NUTRITION
IN A
NUTSHELL

Build Health and Slow Down
the Aging Process

OTHER VITAL HEALTH PUBLISHING/ ENHANCEMENT BOOKS TITLES

Energy For Life: How to Overcome Chronic Fatigue, George Redmon, N.D., Ph.D., 244 pages, 1-890612-14-6, $15.95.

The Cancer Handbook: What's Really Working, edited by Lynne McTaggart, 192 pages, 1-890612-18-9, $12.95.

Wheatgrass: Superfood for a New Millenium, Li Smith, 164 pages, 1-890612-10-3, $10.95.

Stevia Rebaudiana: Nature's Sweet Secret (3rd ed.), David Richard, includes stevia growing information, 80 pages, 1-890612-15-4, $7.95.

Stevia Sweet Recipes: Sugar-Free - Naturally! (2nd ed.), Jeffrey Goettemoeller, 196 pages, 1-890612-13-8, $13.95.

Taste Life! The Organic Choice, Ed. by David Richard and Dorie Byers, R.N., 208 pages, 1-890612-08-1, $12.95.

Lecithin and Health, Frank Orthoefer, Ph.D., 80 pages, 1-890612-03-0, $8.95.

Natural Body Basics: Making Your Own Cosmetics, Dorie Byers, R.N., 88 pages, 0-9652353-0-0, $9.95.

Anoint Yourself With Oil for Radiant Health, David Richard, 56 pages, 1-890612-01-4, $7.95.

My Whole Food ABC's, David Richard and Susan Cavaciuti, 28 color pages, children's, 1-890612-07-3, $8.95.

The Veneration of Life: Through the Disease to the Soul, John Diamond, M.D., 80 pages, 1-890995-14-2, $9.95.

The Way of the Pulse: Drumming With Spirit, John Diamond, M.D., 116 pages, 1-890995-02-9, $13.95.

The Healing Power of Blake: A Distillation, edited by John Diamond, M.D., 180 pages, 1-890995-03-7, $14.95.

The Healer: Heart and Hearth, John Diamond, M.D., 112 pages, 1-890995-22-3, $13.95.

Life Enhancement Through Music, John Diamond, M.D., approx.172 pages, 1-890995-01-0, $14.95.

NUTRITION
IN A
NUTSHELL

*Build Health and Slow Down
the Aging Process*

Bonnie C. Minsky

M.A., M.P.H., C.N.S., L.N.C.

VITAL HEALTH PUBLISHING

Bloomingdale, Illinois

Cover photograph by David Richard
Interior design and production: Woodshed Productions

Nutrition in a Nutshell: *Build Health and Slow Down the Aging Process*

Second Edition Copyright ©2000, Bonnie C. Minsky

Originally published as *Nutrition in a Nutshell: Let's Get Personal–Ten Steps for Building Health and Slowing Down the Aging Process*, © 1999, Bonnie C. Minsky.

Published by: Vital Health Publishing
                  P.O. Box 544
                  Bloomingdale, IL 60108

ISBN: 1-890612-17-0

CONTENTS

Dedication

This book is dedicated to my children
and grandchildren who deserve to live in a world
where healthful eating is the norm instead
of the exception.

In Memoriam

For Eva Carol . . . my mother's early death
encouraged me to ask questions of my healthcare
providers. Now, as a healthcare provider myself,
I will never stop searching for answers.

FOREWORD

In my 20 years plus of interviewing health experts, one of the most rewarding encounters was my conversation with Bonnie C. Minsky. Here was a woman for all ages—menopausal women, children, the elderly. Many of these clients had been plagued with "incurable"conditions until Ms. Minsky detected the cause of their misery. In many cases, the culprit was food sensitivities or unsuspected environmental toxins.

We are so fortunate that this much sought after nutrition authority has taken the time to share her insights and wisdom with us.

> Jane Heimlich, author
> *What Your Doctor Won't Tell You*

As a researcher and educator for over 35 years in the areas of gastrointestinal microecology, probiotics and enzymes, I have long had a concern for the nutritional aspects of health and well-being.

I find your *Nutrition in a Nutshell* is an excellent source of nutrition information that is presented in an easily understandable form, and is exceptionally well researched and documented.

Any family interested in nutritional health should have this book in its house library.

> Khem Shahani, Ph.D.
> *Professor at The Institute of Agriculture and Natural
>   Resources at The University of Nebraska-Lincoln
> World reknowned researcher for the role of acidophilus
>   in nutrition*

Over the past twenty years that I have known Bonnie Minsky, she has had an excellent reputation as a leading Nutrition Couselor. She has been very effective in helping patients who have conditions that can be favorably influenced by dietary changes and nutritional supplementation. Her energy and enthusiasm have complimented her extensive training, knowledge, and experience.

This book should be useful to patients not only with allergies but also a wide variety of other conditions.

Robert W. Boxer, MD.
Fellow of the American Association of Board Certified Allergists, The American Academy of Allergy, Asthma, and Immunology, The American College of Allergy, Asthma, and Immunology, and The Amercian Academy of Environmental Medicine

INTRODUCTION

I have come to believe through many years of research and countless case studies that an individual's ability to resist damage caused by a disease or pathogen is directly related to nutritional balance. This has been the principle I have adhered to for the past 20 years. Nutritional changes are difficult and take time, but the end result is a feeling of total well-being and empowerment.

According to Leo Galland, MD, a key player for the integration of alternative and orthodox medical treatment, "the science of medicine has lost its human face, deformed by the massive technology it has spawned." The depersonalization of healthcare and the dependence of many physicians on laboratory testing instead of listening to the patient's needs has created a disgruntled, frustrated public who will continue to seek answers elsewhere. (Galland, *Four Pillars of Health*, 1997).

I wrote this book in memory of my mother, who died due to medical mismanagement, and for my clients and family who have been frustrated by a medical orthodoxy which refuses to look at the individual first. Instead, it treats patients as just another disease needing "a drug cure."

Drug therapy (which is often necessary for short-term acute conditions) treats the symptoms. Nutritional therapy may take longer, but it offers the potential for correcting the underlying condition by restoring balance, especially for degenerative lifestyle conditions.

Louis Pasteur, the father of microbiology, ironically explained to a group of renowned scientists before he died that, it's not the pathogenic agents (i.e. salmonella, HIV, yeast) we should be concerned about, it's the host. If the host is strong enough, disease cannot thrive.

If I can assist in strengthening the individual (i.e. the host), wellness will usually follow. Besides looking at nutritional imbalance, which is the core of this book, it is important that each person strive for optimum health through finding methods for detoxification, avoiding environmental pollutants, handling stress effectively, adopting a positive attitude, and finding a passion in life. I wish I could personally meet with all of you, my readers, to bring you good health. Unfortunately, because that is not possible, I hope this book can get you started on the long and interesting journey toward optimum health.

⚜ 1 ⚜

Eat to Live, Not Live to Eat

Food and water are essential to life. No living organism can survive very long without them. In fact, if humans had not been able to adapt to changes in the food supply throughout history, our homo sapiens species would have died out. Besides plagues, the most dreaded fear for humans throughout history was famine; they did everything in their power to avoid this dreaded scourge. Fortunately, in the United States of America today, famine is not a common problem. In fact, there are surpluses of many food items. Probably for this reason, a very different fear has set in, especially among affluent Americans. This is the fear of over-eating or gluttony.

Numerous research studies have shown the relationship between chronic overeating and weight gain. Overeating and poor eating habits have been linked to the development of many diseases, including diabetes, cancer, and heart disease (for more detailed information, see Chapter #9). Preliminary animal studies have also indicated that calorie restriction slows down the aging process. Thus, it is realistic that we should restrict our portions of various food items (which will be outlined in future chapters), avoid addictions to any single food (i.e. sugar) or group of foods (i.e. carbohydrates), and eat a wide variety of foods to sustain life. These lifestyle habits should be gradual changes that build muscle, burn fat and build health. Eating food for sustenance should be pleasurable; eating should not invoke fear.

Unfortunately common sense often falls by the wayside. Many Americans, especially teenage girls and young women, believe that all food can be potentially harmful. Their fear of food has reached epidemic proportions, and

1

often manifests itself in the form of anorexia nervosa (self-imposed starvation) or bulimia (eating large quantities of food, then purging). According to Michelle Stacey's recent book, entitled *Consumed*, people living in countries where food is overabundant, such as in the United States, are stressed out over the moral, physical, and spiritual corruption that comes from the fat, cholesterol, sugar, salt, or any of the hundreds of mysterious additives in their diets. Stacey's message is that rather than looking for magical salvation in the supermarkets and health-food stores, learn to *live in close harmony with our food; rather than to struggle against it, consider it a source of life, not death.*

Real food should be enjoyed, loved, and treated as a basic life instinct. If there is to be any consciousness-raising, (not fear), related to food, it should focus on protecting our food supply from unnecessary and unsafe food handling practices, harmful food additives, and chemical pesticides (see Chapters #2 and #3 for detailed information). Taking steps to ensure safe foods for all Americans should empower us, not create fear. The most basic concept of **eating to live** means that we should not harbor obsessions about food by overeating, undereating, or refusing to eat at all. Since the beginning of human existence, it has been proven that if we eat real food in moderation, our bodies have the ability to build muscle, burn fat, build health, and slow down the aging process. In the next few chapters, the steps for accomplishing these goals successfully will be described in detail.

Begin right now by savoring the wonderful tastes, smells, and varieties of **real** food. Celebrate food because it gives us the energy not only to sustain life, but also to accomplish the World Health Organization's definition of health, which is *optimum physical, mental, emotional, and social well-being.*

Personal Case Study #1

Gina B, a small, painfully thin 5´4, 96 lb. twenty-five year old, had struggled with anorexia nervosa or bulimia since the age of 11. Both of her obese parents had frightened her into thinking that fats were her enemy and the fewer calories she ingested the healthier and thinner she would be. Even though she was a super athlete, sometimes practicing or participating in a sporting event for three hours or more daily, she counted her pretzels, rice cakes and cereal individually so that she would not overdo her calorie intake. She also refused to take in more than 10 grams of fat daily. She had daily headaches and stomach pains which no one paid attention to until she fainted during a soccer match. A doctor ran a blood test to find that her electrolytes were unbalanced. Her iron, total cholesterol and triglycerides were very low, which can be an indication of anemia and malnutrition.

When I met with her eight years later, her symptoms were unchanged. The fear in her pale eyes was evident. Her fear was not of being unhealthy, but fear that I might force her to eat more calories and fats which would force her to gain weight. I always determine zinc status with clients who have eating disorders. Her zinc level was so low that she was not getting the appropriate hunger signal. When we supplemented with zinc and other nutrients and gave her evidence of her ability to eat to build muscle while burning fat, she was willing to try new foods one baby step at a time. She also received psychological counseling from a well-respected eating disorders specialist.

Today, Gina is a vibrant, athletic-looking young woman who is proud of her muscular 120 lb., 5´4 body. She has become a public health nutritionist working in a health club with young women who she says are "clueless about healthy eating."

~❦ 2 ❦~

Eat Real Food

Many health professionals profess the theory that there are no bad foods and that as long as unhealthy foods are consumed on an occasional basis, they are fine. It is true that all foods that provide **nutrients** (proteins, carbohydrates, fats, trace vitamins/minerals, water, and enzymes) are safe, even if they sometimes contain too much or too little of any one substance. When these types of nutrient-dense foods are eaten, the human body knows how to break them down, digest and absorb them, and utilize them at the cellular level. Even a piece of chocolate cake made with real eggs, butter, milk, cocoa powder, pure maple syrup, and flour would be acceptable in moderation because your body is familiar with all of the ingredients. Unfortunately, thousands of the "so-called foods" we see in the marketplace today are merely **fake** foods (i.e. they have nothing to nourish life). That delicious piece of homemade chocolate cake will get stale and grow bacteria if not eaten within a few days. On the other hand, a heavily processed brand-name cupcake (such as the one I currently have in my possession) that has grown no bacteria and still smells like chocolate after 17 years cannot be classified as a food. If mold won't feed on it, why should we?

A real food should grow moldy or get rotten (just be sure to eat it before it does get rotten). If it doesn't grow moldy or get rotten, we can't really classify it as a food. Some of these wonders of technology include soft drinks, hard candy, popsicles, sugar substitutes, and non-dairy creamers. There are literally thousands of them sold in our grocery stores.

5

I would like to further define a **fake** food as 1) a product manufactured with a host of man-made chemicals 2) processed by unsafe methods (i.e. hydrogenation of fats in the manufacture of most margarines), or 3) a product so overly processed that it bears little, if any, resemblance to its natural state. Our bodies have had thousands or even hundreds of thousands of years to genetically adapt to certain plant and animal foods, but we have had a mere fifty years to attempt adaptation to chemically-laden, over-processed products. This is why degenerative diseases are skyrocketing and why Americans are getting heavier in spite of all of our lowfat "diet" foods. The more fake foods we consume, the sicker and heavier we will become as a population.

Food additives, as commonly used in the international food supply, are not always harmful. Some, in fact, are nutrients, chemicals found in nature, or harmless substances. However, many food additives are man-made, contain naturally occurring toxins, or are chemically altered from their original state. Thus, they may pose serious health risks including rashes, hyperkinetic behavior, edema, breathing problems, and even death. TABLE I: (Collected Reports of Adverse Reactions to MSG and Aspartame) and TABLE II: (Food Additives—Friends or Foes) specifically mentions names and adverse reactions to just some of the hundreds of food additives used by manufacturers to flavor, preserve, or color processed foods.

Two of the most widely used and most dangerous food additives are Monosodium Glutamate (MSG) and Aspartame (Nutrasweet®/Equal®). As seen in Table I, almost one-half of all people who were tested for reactions to these two substances, showed symptoms. Although both substances are derived from natural amino acids, the chemical alteration from their naturally occurring state (in protein-rich foods) into the flavor enhancer, MSG, and the sugar substitute, Aspartame, totally changes their molecular structures and renders them neurotoxic.

Monosodium Glutamate (see Table I) is a particularly dangerous neurotoxin, according to Russell Blaylock, M. D. (Blaylock, *Excitotoxins: The Taste that Kills*, 1994). Because it blocks Vitamin B-6 and the mineral magnesium, it blatantly affects serotonin balance in the brain and kills neurons. The actual manufacture of MSG is also highly suspect. According to Blaylock, to make hydrolyzed protein (a form of MSG), you take *junk vegetables unfit for sale, with high amounts of glutamate, boiled in a vat of acid, and neutralized with caustic soda. This brown sludge becomes dried, brown powder high in glutamate, aspartate and cystoic acid which converts in the body to cysteine, another excitotoxin.* This is not a very appetizing picture. Besides the excitotoxic effect of hydrolyzed protein, many people are allergic to the corn, soy, or wheat proteins from which it is derived. Just recently, the Food and Drug Administration demanded that all products containing hydrolyzed protein must be labeled by source.

Aspartame (Nutrasweet®/Equal®), for a short time, appeared to be the perfect sugar substitute. It is derived from two amino acids (aspartic acid and phenylalanine), so it is touted as being natural. It is also 200 times sweeter than sugar and non-caloric. It has become a staple in dietetic foods and is also highly recommended, even by the medical profession, for diabetics who must limit consumption of carbohydrates. Parents are even giving it to very young children in the hopes of preventing dental caries from excess sugar or obesity from too many simple sugar calories. Unfortunately, the longer it has been used, the more problems researchers and consumers have uncovered from its use. Aspartame has been found to overexcite the brain (Blaylock, *Excitotoxins: The Taste that Kills*), which overstimulates and kills brain cells. As with MSG, the important nutrients B-6 and magnesium are also depleted. The most serious reactions to aspartame (as reported in Table I) include convulsions, vision problems, headaches, memory loss, depression, dizziness, behavioral changes, insomnia, skin rashes, bloating, and weight gain. Children react more violently to aspartame because of their lower body weight and rapid brain cell growth. Many children consume far more than the tested "safety" level.

There is a great risk to a child whose mother consumes aspartame while pregnant. Because it contains a concentrated amount of phenylalanine, aspartame may contribute to the genetic disorder, PKU. If a pregnant woman happens to be an unknown carrier of PKU, her unborn child will be at far greater risk for developing more serious complications of this disorder. PKU warnings must be present for every product containing aspartame.

Nutrasweet® has been a dismal failure as a weight loss substance. In numerous studies of thousands of men and women consuming this sugar substitute, as cited by Dr. Russell Blaylock, weight gain was more likely to occur among Nutrasweet® users. Just look around you. How many thin people do you see consuming diet soft drinks?

As a practicing nutrition counselor, I have personally witnessed thousands of adverse reactions to aspartame and MSG. Bloating and/or weight gain have occurred among most of the users I have encountered. Obesity is also a common problem for individuals consuming both substances, even among those who are on restricted calorie diets. The most serious reactions I have seen have been extreme memory loss to a surgeon consuming seven cans of diet soft drinks daily (he had to stop performing surgery) and classic multiple sclerosis symptoms to a college student who consumed six diet soft drinks and copious diet foods (laden with aspartame or MSG). Fortunately, both of these individuals had complete reversal of symptoms when the offending substances were avoided for at least one month.

Artificial food colorings, derived from coal tar, are food additives that cause severe reactions to sensitive individuals. F. D. & C. Yellow #5 (tartrazine), in particular, must be listed on all food labels that contain it because of severe allergic reactions. Hyperkinetic behavior, rash, edema, and even anaphylactic shock have occurred when small amounts of this substance are consumed. Red Dye #40, which has been banned in all new food products and medications, has been shown to cause severe bladder irritation and even bladder cancer if consumed regularly.

In the last ten years, there has been an alarming increase in Attention Deficit Disorder (ADD), hyperkinetic behavior, and learning disabilities among American children. In 1990, 750,000 children were diagnosed with ADD. In 1995, that figure rose to almost 4,000,000. Most of these children are prescribed the drug, Ritalin (which is classified as an amphetamine). Ritalin's common side effects are poor appetite and growth retardation. During the withdrawal stages (which are common on weekends and when school is not in session), more serious reactions, including violent or aggressive behavior and even suicide, have been reported. The sad fact is that most hyperactive behavior and attention deficit disorder can be reversed by a high protein, nutrient-dense diet devoid of harmful additives. In countries where this type of diet is the norm, these problems are virtually non-existent.

Be aware that most food manufacturers have a host of options to flavor, preserve, or color the items they send to the marketplace. They often choose the potentially harmful additives over the safe ones because they save a few pennies (i.e. Beta Carotene costs more to color a food than does a yellow coal tar dye such as Yellow #5 or #6). If consumers refuse to purchase foods made with harmful additives, food manufacturers will be forced to either change the product or go out of business. A wonderful example of consumer power is a large cereal company that supplied thousands of boxes of a rice cereal to the New York Public School system. The buyer for the city-wide breakfast program told the company they would have to find another supplier if the BHA and BHT were not removed from their cereal. Not only did this mega-corporation remove these preservatives promptly from the cereal shipped to the New York City Public Schools, but they removed them in all of their cereals. This way the public had safer food and the cereal company sold more cereal.

To see how **real** your present diet truly is, make a checklist of all of the foods in your kitchen that contain two or more "Foe" additives (listed in Table II). Separate these items from the foods that have no harmful additives (if the total product has under 300 mg. of salt or 3 gm. or less of sugar, it doesn't have to be listed as a "Foe" additive). If you're heavy on the "Foe" side, you know that you'll need to make some major dietary changes. To make it easier for you to accomplish this, we've included your own personal "Natural Foods Shopping Tour" list of additive-free brand name foods (see Appendix B).

You should be suspicious of any complicated chemical process that alters your food. Mechanical food processes are much safer because they don't cause nutrient depletion or molecular structure changes in most cases. For instance, extra virgin olive oil is the mechanical first pressing of olives. This form of olive oil is a rich source of monounsaturated fat. Its nutritional benefits have not been altered. On the other hand, the process often used to decaffeinate coffee uses the dangerous chemical, methylene chloride (see Table II; Food Additives: Friends or Foes?). Coffee companies have the option of using a safe, water process instead. If the U. S. Food and Drug Administration would ban some of these harmful substances (see more detailed information in Chapter #3), the public wouldn't need a biochemistry degree to figure out what foods are fit for human consumption.

Personal Case Study #2

Bryan O. was an 8 year old, skinny, blue-eyed blond who was so hyperkinetic that he could not sit in my office long enough to draw a picture (my "Draw a Man" test) of himself. He touched and moved all of my food displays to the point of distraction. His mother finally asked him to play outdoors, whereupon he ran down a hill into a muddy creek. The Ritalin prescribed by his pediatrician made him either "zombie-like" when he took it or a self-destructive tyrant when he went off of it during holiday vacations. The day before our Thanksgiving holiday appointment, he had jumped off a neighbor's roof onto their car, denting it. The angry neighbors banned Bryan from their property until he could prove that he was able to control himself. His mother cried openly in my office because she had seen glimpses of a sweet, intelligent, calm young man on rare occasions and that's the Bryan she refused to stop searching for. I asked her what his favorite foods were and her immediate response was Popsicles, hard candy, and high-sugared cereals. He really went for "bright colors." We decided to put him on a two week elimination diet avoiding common allergens and food additives. We discovered a minor corn allergy which affected his concentration, but his worst reactions were to FD&C Yellow #5, Red Dye #40 and Caramel Color. These petrochemical substances turned his behavior "animalistic." His cognitive function during these times was replaced by a brain stem "fight or flight" existence.

Bryan was so relieved to realize that chemicals caused his bizarre, animalistic, uncontrolled behavior that he avoided them completely. He now is totally off of Ritalin and is a friendly, well-adjusted child.

TABLE I

Collected Reports of Adverse Reactions to MSG and Aspartame

Ingestion of monosodium glutamate (MSG) is known to produce a variety of adverse reactions in certain people. These reactions, although seemingly dissimilar, are no more diverse than the reactions found as side effects of certain neurological drugs. We do not know why certain people experience reactions and others do not. We do not know whether MSG "causes" the condition underlying the reaction, or whether the underlying condition is simply aggravated by the ingestion of MSG. We only know that the following are sometimes caused or exacerbated by ingestion of MSG. We also know that manufactured glutamate in all of its other forms (hydrolyzed protein, sodium caseinate, autolyzed yeast, etc.), can bring on these same adverse reactions in MSG sensitive persons.

Aspartame poses similar reactions to MSG, especially when consumed in high-acid, protein-deficient drinks.

Cardiac
Extreme drop in blood pressure
Rapid heartbeat (tachycardia)
Angina
Arrhythmias

Circulatory
Swelling

Muscular
Flu-like achiness
Joint pain
Stiffness

Respiratory
Asthma, Shortness of breath
Chest pain
Runny nose, Sneezing

Skin
Hives or rash
Mouth lesions
Temporary tightness or partial
    paralysis
Numbness or tingling of the skin
Flushing
Extreme dryness of the mouth

Gastrointestinal
Nausea/vomiting
Stomach cramps
Irritable bowel
Bloating
Diarrhea

Neurological
Depression
Anxiety
Dizziness
Panic attacks
Light-headedness
Hyperactivity
Loss of balance
Lethargy
Slurred speech
Sleepiness
Disorientation
Insomnia
Mental confusion
Behavioral problems in children
Migraine and other headaches

Visual
Blurred Vision
Difficulty in focusing

*In addition, research has implicated glutamate in diseases that include the following:

Alzheimer's disease	Huntington's disease
Amotrophic lateral sclerosis (ALS)	Parkinson's disease
Epilepsy	Schizophrenia

Hidden Sources of MSG

The following are food label descriptors that are always or often associated with the presence of MSG in food products:

Monosodium glutamate	Autolyzed yeast
Hydrolyzed protein	Textured protein
Sodium caseinate	Calcium caseinate
Yeast extract	Yeast food
Yeast nutrient	

ASPARTAME (NUTRASWEET®): IS IT SAFE?

Aspartame (Nutrasweet®) has become the most popular low-calorie sweetener in the world since its controversial approval in 1981. Two hundred million people are consuming it, including one hundred million adults. But there is a problem: more than 80% of the complaints about foods and additives received by the FDA involved Aspartame. The Centers for Disease Control have reported over 6,000 adverse reactions including convulsions, vision problems, headache, memory loss, depression, dizziness, behavioral changes, insomnia, skin rashes, bloating, and weight gain.

COLLECTED REPORTS OF ADVERSE REACTIONS COMPARING ASPARTAME WITH MSG

The following table lists the percentages of the human population reacting to MSG and Aspartame and is categorized according to symptoms.

	Percent of all complaints for	
Symptoms	**MSG ***	**Aspartame ** **
Headache	21.0	19.3
Vomiting and nausea	8.7	6.6
Abdominal pain and cramps	4.6	4.9
Fatigue, weakness	3.2	2.8
Sleep problems	2.8	2.6
Change in vision	2.7	3.4
Change in activity level	1.6	1.3
Total Complaints	**44.6**	**40.9**

*LSRO/FASEB, 1993   **Tollefson, 1988

Please Note: As you can see from the similarity in reactions, MSG and NutraSweet® behave almost the same way in the human brain. Aspartic Acid, found in NutraSweet® is a neurotoxic amino acid, as is glutamic acid, MSG. Why are these food additives still allowed in our food supply when almost half of the population reacts to them?

Sources:

Blaylock, Russell, M.D. *Excitotoxins: The Taste that Kills.* Health Press: Santa Fe, 1994.

Centers for Disease Control, Atlanta, Georgia.

No MSG (consumer group) www.truthinlabeling.org

Roberts, H.J., M.D. *Sweetener Dearest,, Bittersweet Vignettes About Aspartame* (Nutrasweet®). Sunshine Centennial Press, 1992.

Schwartz, George R., M.D. *In Bad Taste: The MSG Syndrome.* Health Press, Sante Fe, 1990.

TABLE II
FOOD ADDITIVES: FRIENDS OR FOES?

The food additives listed below are considered "Friends" if they cause few, if any, side effects. Additives are considered "Foes" if they have been poorly tested, have been proven harmful, or may be harmful to human health if used in large quantities. Many harmful additives now being used have safer substitutes, many of which are listed below. An educated consumer will always ask the following question: Are the food additives in this particular product there for my safety or to increase corporate profits?

FRIENDS

1. **Alpha Tocopherol** (Vitamin E)—prevents oils from getting rancid; preservative
2. **Annatto** (extracted from annatto tree)—used as a vegetable dye and a spice flavoring; no known toxicity
3. **Ascorbic Acid** (Vitamin C)—helps maintain the red color of meat; used as a preservative and to prevent the formation of nitrosamines
4. **Beta Carotene** (converts to Vitamin A)—used as a yellow food coloring and nutrient
5. **Calcium** (or Sodium) Propionate—prevents mold growth on bread and rolls; the calcium is a nutrient; no toxicity
6. **Citric Acid** (found abundantly in nature— especially in fruits & berries)—used to give a tart flavoring and as an antioxidant
7. **EDTA**—a chelating agent that traps metal impurities which might promote rancidity or contamination of foods
8. **Ferrous Gluconate** (Iron)—a nutrient used as a source of iron and as a black coloring
9. **Fumaric Acid**—(essential to vegetable and animal tissue respiration)— an ideal source of tartness and acidity in dry food products
10. **Gelatin**—(protein from animal bones)— used as a thickening agent

11. **Glycerin/Glycerol**—(forms the backbone of fat & oil molecules)—used to maintain water content in food
12. **Gums**—(derived from natural sources such guar, locust, and arabic) —used as thickening agents and stabilizers
13. **Lactic Acid**—(occurs in all living organisms) used to inhibit spoilage and to balance acidity
14. **Lecithin**—(source of valuable nutrient—choline)—used as an emulsifier, antioxidant, & preventative for oil spattering
15. **Mannitol**—(found naturally in plants); used as a sweetener and texturizer
16. **Mono & Diglycerides**—softening and emulsifying agents for many processed foods
17. **Sorbic Acid**—(occurs naturally in berries of the mountain ash); may be a safe replacement for sodium nitrate but needs tests; protects against molds and other fungi
18. **Sorbitol**—(occurs naturally in fruits and berries, also a close relative of sugars)—used as a sweetener, thickening agent, and moisture retainer; does not cause blood sugar to increase rapidly; absorbed slowly; LARGE AMOUNTS MAY CAUSE DIARRHEA
19. **Starch, Modified Starch**—(major component of flour, potatoes, & corn)—used as a thickening agent
20. **Tumeric**—(derived from an East Indian herb)—used as a yellow food coloring and flavoring; no known toxicity
21. **Vanillin, Ethyl Vanillin**—(used as a substitute for the vanilla bean) —produced cheaply in the factory; appears to be safe

QUESTIONABLE ADDITIVES

1. **Caffeine**—stimulant drug that has adverse effects in large quantities, but in small amount helps mental clarity; AVOID IF CAFFEINE SENSITIVE

2. **Fructose**—a naturally occurring sugar found in many fruits and honey but prepared commercially in the United States from corn; absorbed more slowly than most sugars so may be acceptable for those suffering from blood sugar imbalances; excess amounts create nutrient deficiencies; avoid if corn sensitive

3. **Lactose (Milk Sugar)**—used commercially as a sweetener; at least 60% of the adult world population has trouble digesting milk sugar; if you experience gas, bloating, and/or diarrhea from milk, AVOID LACTOSE AS AN ADDITIVE

4. **Polysorbate 60**—used as an emulsifier and flavor dispersing agent in shortening and edible oils; the FDA has asked for further study to prove safety

5. **Potassium Sorbate**—a preservative used to inhibit mold and other fungi; low oral toxicity, but may cause a mild skin irritation among sensitive individuals

6. **Salt (Sodium Chloride)**—although an essential mineral, it is over-used in processed foods and may increase the risk of high blood pressure, stroke, and edema; the average intake should be between 1,100-3,300 mg. daily

7. **Sodium Benzoate**—prevents the growth of microorganisms primarly in acidic foods; used in a wide variety of foods and medications; it can cause intestinal upset urticaria, and angioedema in sensitive individuals (especially if aspirin sensitive)

Foes

1. **BST (Bovine Growth Hormone)**—may affect human health growth patterns and hormone balance; milk from BST cows has higher antibiotic residues; may be carcinogenic
2. **Antibiotics and Hormones**—used abundantly in animal feed; residues often appear in chicken, eggs, meat, and milk; cause antibiotic resistant pathogens
3. **Artificial Food Colorings**—most harmful are Yellow No. 5, Yellow No. 6, and Red No. 40; may cause serious allergic reactions
4. **Artificial Food Flavorings**—used almost entirely in "junk" foods & is a sure indication that the "real" thing has been left out
5. **Aspartame (Nutrasweet®)**—a compound of 2 amino acids; must be avoided by persons with PKU; safety in question due to large amounts used in nutrient-poor foods and quality of testing; noted side effects are dizziness, headaches, blurred vision, and seizures; NEEDS MORE TESTS
6. **Autolyzed Yeast**—see "Monosodium Glutamate"
7. **BHA, BHT**— preservatives that retard rancidity & oxidation; some studies suggest harmful effects; safer substitutes exist; needs more tests
8. **Caffeine**—stimulant drug that can have adverse effects in large quantities
9. **Corn Sugar & Corn Syrup**—no nutritional values; "empty" calories; common allergens
10. **Hydrogenated Vegetable Oil**—the by-product of chemical process that converts oils into semi-solids which causes them to become more saturated (used in many margarines & shortenings); may cause plaque to form on artery walls
11. **Hydrolyzed Vegetable Protein**—see "Monosodium Glutamate"
12. **Methylene Chloride**—used to decaffeinate coffee; causes cancer in animals; good substitutes are water process or ethyl acetate decaf coffees including High Point, Folgers, Taster's Choice, Marager Gold and Nescafe
13. **Monosodium Glutamate (MSG)**—This animal glutamic acid and its derivatives such as autolyzed yeast and Hydrolyzed Vegetable Protein (HVP) cause very unpleasant side effects for those sensitive to them; some studies suggest that they destroy nerve cells in the brain; should not be consumed by infants & toddlers

14. **Phosphoric Acid**—not usually toxic, but the widespread use in foods & drinks has led to mineral depletion (especially calcium); most Americans consume too much phosphorous
15. **Propyl Gallate**—used as an antioxidant (usually with BHA & BHT); may cause cancer
16. **Quinine**—very poorly tested as a flavoring; causes reactions in sensitive individuals; used as a drug to treat malaria
17. **Saccharin**—350 times sweeter than sugar; large amounts have been shown to cause cancer in animals; banned in Canada & FDA proposed a ban in 1977
18. **Sodium Nitrate & Nitrite**—can lead to the formation of nitrosamines which can cause cancer; prevents growth of bacteria in meats & gives cured meat its red color
19. **Invert Sugar**—sweeter than sucrose; provides only empty calories
20. **Sugar**—contains only "empty" calories & makes up about 1/4–1/6 of the American diet; much of it is hidden in processed foods; the more processed the sugar, the worse it is.
21. **Sulfites (Sulfur Dioxide, Sodium Bisulfite)**—prevent discoloration of fruits & vegetables; prevent bacterial growth in wine; destroys Vitamin B-1; can cause serious allergic reactions . . . even death!

≈ 3 ≈

Eat Safe Food and Drink Safe Water

Most Americans take food safety for granted. We assume that because we have governmental protection and intervention practices that oversee our food and water supplies, that we are protected from pesticides and contamination. This couldn't be farther from the truth. Presently, our Food and Drug Administration only tests new chemical substances for cancer. Our own U.S. Congress and Office of Technology Assessment (OTA) wrote an eye-opening book in 1990 entitled *Neurotoxicity* (U.S. Government Printing Office), in which they urged the Food and Drug Administration to test the thousands of chemicals used regularly in our food and water supplies for neurotoxicity. Congress felt very strongly that the many independent studies that reported serious adverse effects from chemicals and pesticides have been virtually ignored by the FDA, whose job it is to protect the public from harmful foods, drugs, and chemicals. But when politics and revolving door practices occur among top FDA officials, the public's safety often will be short-changed. It is time for the FDA to acknowledge and begin acting upon the concerns of the OTA, Congress and the American Public.

Fortunately, the U.S. Public is demanding chemical and pesticide-free foods. Organic farming has skyrocketed in this country so much so that the demand for organically grown and organically processed foods has sometime outweighed the supply. As more and more consumers insist upon buying only organically grown produce and free-range animal protein, farmers will increasingly switch to organic farming methods.

Probably the most serious health risk to our food supply today is the addition of **antibiotics** to animal feed and injections given to our poultry, dairy cows, and steers (beef). The hormones and antibiotic residues are consumed every time we eat chicken, eggs, dairy products, or beef that are not free-range or organic. One of the major reasons that U.S. citizens are losing the war against pneumonia, strep, tuberculosis, salmonella, and many other life-threatening illnesses is due to the fact that we have developed antibiotic resistant strains of the organisms that cause these illnesses. According to *The Kellogg Report* (Joseph Beasley, M. D., The Institute of Health Policy and Practices, 1989), even moderate use of antibiotics in animal feed can result in the development of antibiotic resistance in animal bacteria with the subsequent transfer of that resistance to human bacteria. A perfect example of pathogen resistance was a serious outbreak of salmonella in the milk supplied to Chicago area stores in the late 1980s. The milk contained an antibiotic-resistant strain of salmonella, which made the problem more difficult to treat. A few individuals who were given antibiotics actually died because the antibiotics killed their healthy intestinal flora instead of killing the salmonella.

Contamination from **pathogens** in food has become such a serious problem in the United States today that there is a national outcry for safer food. Outbreaks of salmonella, shigella, e. coli, giardia, and botulism have become almost as widespread as the common cold. The severity of food poisoning depends upon which bacteria are involved, how much is ingested, and the strength of the host (i.e. the human who ingested the pathogen) to defend against it (see TABLE I for a list of the most common pathogens and what to do about them). Most of these pathogens have been around for thousands of years. The reason they are posing such a great threat to human health in the U.S. today is because they have become "superbugs." They resist most of the drugs with which we have to treat them, and we have done a great job in killing our healthy intestinal flora (which is our best protection against them). There are many ways we can protect ourselves from ingesting these pathogens (see

TABLE II). Besides avoidance through strict safety measures, we can provide ourselves with excellent protection by consuming Lactobacillus Acidophilus and/or Bifidus (either in an active-culture organic yogurt or in powder/capsule form) on a regular basis. In fact, when I recommend these flora to my clients suffering from salmonella, their health improves rapidly.

Another serious food contamination problem, that often goes unrecognized, is the addition of growth hormones to animal feed. These **growth hormones** are "beefing" us up and playing havoc with our own hormone balance. In fact, several studies have linked constant ingestion of hormone residues in animal feed to hormonal (particularly of the breast) cancers. Now the FDA has even approved the genetically engineered bovine growth hormone (BST) to increase milk production in cows. The long-term effects are unknown, but the animal studies used to prove its safety were either flawed or falsified, according to Dr. Samuel Epstein of The University of Illinois at Chicago School of Public Health and an expert in the environmental causes of cancer. Dr. Epstein has repeatedly expressed concern that BST is causing a surge in rapidly growing hormonal and brain cancers, as all of the preliminary animal studies indicated. Until recently, the European Common Market would not import any animal foods from The United States unless they were certified hormone-free. Most European countries have banned the use of hormones in their animal feed. The United Nations recently banned imported animal foods from the United States unless they are certified hormone-free. What have they learned that American farmers and chemical companies won't acknowledge?

For total safety, the American public should only consume animal proteins (particularly chicken, eggs, beef and dairy products) that are certified organic, free-range, or imported. The law of supply and demand is our best protection when food safety is involved. If consumers refuse to buy contaminated, hormone and antibiotic laced foods, agribusiness will stop producing these items.

Besides contamination of food, **water contamination** is becoming a more serious problem in the United States, even with good water filtration methods. Various pathogens have become resistant to the chlorine and fluoride used to kill them, making them "superbugs" and thus, more difficult to destroy. Lead, copper, and other heavy metals are also causing serious problems in many city water pipes, which affect brain activity, especially among children. Even the chlorine and fluoride added to water to supposedly benefit human health have also been shown to suppress the immune system and cause toxic reactions among sensitive individuals. For instance, in a recent study conducted by the California Department of Health Services, it was found that pregnant women who consumed large amounts of chlorinated tap water raised their risk of miscarriages significantly.

Safe water is essential to human health. Probably the safest water to drink in the United States today is natural spring water which has been obtained from springs that bubble up from the ground in areas where the ground water is unpolluted. Spring water abounds with naturally occurring minerals. The next safest water is distilled, which is processed by heating water and evaporating the steam. This procedure removes all impurities and toxins. However, it also eliminates the important trace minerals.

If you live in an area with a high mineral content water (often termed "hard water"), it is usually healthiest and most cost-effective to use a reverse osmosis carbon filter for all drinking water (and ideally for bath water also). Research has indicated that geographical areas containing "hard water" show fewer pockets of heart disease and osteoporosis, most presumably from constant consumption of trace minerals. Softened water, especially if softened with sodium, is not recommended for drinking water or for watering plants because the high level of sodium may cause edema, high blood pressure and imbalanced electrolytes in humans and can cause plants to dry out and die. Our bodies are made up of about 70% water; it's just common sense that we should replace our body's water stores with only the best!

Personal Case Study #3

Al S. was a 22 year old college student who had to drop out of college due to his chronic diarrhea and lethargy. Within the last 18 months he had lost 52 pounds from his already lanky 6´3 frame and had become despondent. He had been to 11 different doctors, been on six different diets and had most recently been existing on buffalo meat, sweet potatoes and water (the only foods that did not cause instant pain or diarrhea). He informed me that I was his last hope.

The first question I asked was, "Have you been out of the country within the last two years?" He had traveled throughout the Middle East, drank water directly out of streams in Israel and had gotten sick several times during a summer odyssey several months before. He informed me that his doctors had tested him several times for parasites, but only once each time. I explained that it often takes three to four cultures, days apart, to detect an active parasite. Because he had suffered so much already, I decided to take a drastic step of recommending herbal, broad-spectrum, parasite-fighting preparations while adding probiotics (acidophilus and bifidus) to restore healthy flora. As he improved symptomatically we were able to add over 15 foods that did not cause adverse reactions.

Three months after our first visit, Al called me in hysteria to ask what he should do about a 12 foot "snake" he had just eliminated with a bowel movement. I told him to bring it to the local hospital for identification. It turned out to be a large tapeworm that may still be on display in one of our local hospitals. The addition of the herbal formulas and probiotics had created an undesirable environment for the organism which dislodged from Al's intestinal walls. The good news is that Al can now eat everything and his former weight and college life have been restored.

TABLE I
FOOD SAFETY – FOOD POISONING

Bacteria	Sources	Prevention	Symptoms	Onset	Recovery
Camphylo-bacteria	Raw Chicken, undercooked meat, poultry, shellfish, un-treated water & unpasteurized milk	Avoid undercooked meat & shellfish. Avoid water from streams, lakes & rivers unless it's been filtered. Avoid unpasteurized milk	Diarrhea, stomach pain, nausea, & vomiting	2-10 days after eating	up to 10 days
Salmonella	Undercooked or improperly refrigerated meat, poultry, stuffing, eggs, unpasteurized milk	Never eat raw or undercooked fish or meat. Never eat raw eggs or milk unless they have been pasteurized	Diarrhea, headache, abdominal pain, fever, chills, and vomiting	6-48 hours after eating	usually in 2-4 days
Clostridium perfringens	Undercooked meat & poultry, foods left out too long	This microorganism grows rapidly in temps. of up to 125 degrees. Thus, food left out too long on steam tables for buffets may allow it to grow. Cooked foods must be kept at temps. higher than 140 degrees or lower than 40 degrees to avoid contamination	Diarrhea & gas pains	8-24 hours	usually in 2-4 days

Staphylococcus aureus	Deli salads like egg & potato, custards, cream filled desserts & dairy products	Contamination by this organism accounts for about 20% of food borne illness in the U.S. Avoiding dairy products, creamy salads, cream fillings, and custards that have been left out over 15 minutes may prevent contamination	Cramps, vomiting, diarrhea	30 minutes to 8 hours	usually in 1 day
Botulism toxin	Home-canned foods or damaged cans & containers of low-acid foods & food kept in conditions where oxygen is limited	Never buy a product in a dented can. Keep home-processed canned goods air tight before use	Double vision, dry mouth, impaired speech & difficulty breathing	12 to 72 hours	Can be fatal if not treated immediately
E. Coli 0157:H7	Raw or undercooked meat, especially raw hamburger; it has also been found in cider and uncooked salami	Cook meat completely through (no pink). Never eat raw meats like steak tartare.	Only a few bacteria can cause symptoms of nausea, vomiting, and dehydration, which can be life-threatening to young children and the elderly	Usually 6-48 hours after eating	up to 2 weeks

Treatment and source information follows on the next page.

Treatment: If you eat contaminated foods and begin to have flu-like symptoms, stop all solid food and drink plenty of water, diluted fruit juice, flat ginger ale, rest and be alert for possible dehydration. If symptoms are severe or persist for more than 12 hours, particularly if you are very young or old or have a chronic illness, seek medical attention. If you are unable to keep fluids down, you may be given an I.V.

Sources:
Terry Corr, office manager, American Seafood Institute, 1-800 EAT-FISH
Bessie Berry, supervisor, USDA Meat and Poultry Hotline
Fighting Back—How to Protect Yourself Against the 'Food Bug' and *Report Food Poisoning Hazards* (M & C, $15.95) by Michael H. Doom, registered environmental health specialist
Poisoned Food? (Glouchester, $12.40) by Tim Lobstein
American Public Health Association, Washington, D.C.

TABLE II
FOOD SAFETY SURVIVAL GUIDE
Handling Food in the Home:
The majority of food-borne illnesses are caused by improper food handling at home each year, and each year in the U.S. about 9,000 people die as a result of food poisoning.

General Handling
Utensils: Consider using an acrylic cutting board if possible, since scratches and cuts in the wood boards can hide bacteria and food particles. Wood boards can be sanitized with chlorine bleach and water. Acrylic cutting boards can also be cleaned in your dishwasher.

Work with only one perishable food at a time. Wash the board and utensils with hot, soapy water between uses.

Cooking Tips
Use a thermometer to ensure that meat and poultry are fully cooked. Put the thermometer in the thickest part of the meat, avoiding fat and bone. Bacteria is killed when meat reaches 160 degrees Fahrenheit; poultry, 180 degrees or higher.

Don't interrupt cooking by starting the job and then finishing the rest later. Partially-cooked food can be warm enough to encourage bacterial growth.

Food Storage
- Chill leftovers as soon as possible and at least within two hours of eating.
- Thaw frozen foods in the refrigerator, by placing the frozen package in a watertight plastic bag in cold water and replacing the water often.
- To protect other foods from germ-carrying meat juices, put meats in separate plastic bags at the store and then on plates before refrigerating.
- Foods that start out cold, such as opened lunch meats, should be wrapped in plastic or aluminum foil before storing.
- To cool hot foods, run cold water over sealed containers before refrigerating so the food reaches ideal storage temperature sooner.

- Store eggs inside the refrigerator compartment, not on the door compartment, because eggs need to be kept cold and often the door is not as cold as the rest of the refrigerator.
- Freezing will stop bacterial growth in certain foods, but only extreme temperatures when cooking will kill bacteria.
- Refrigerator should be set to 40 degrees or below and the freezer should be kept at 10 degrees or below. Verify temperatures with a thermometer.

Brown Bag Lunch Tips

Perishable meats or dairy products should be frozen (they'll defrost by lunch); or a frozen drink (in paper or plastic) should be added to the sealed bag.

Usage Dates to Ensure Freshness

FOOD	REFRIGERATOR	FREEZER
Poultry		
Uncooked	1-2 days	9 months
Cooked	3-4 days	4-6 months
Meat		
All fresh meats		
(steaks, chops & roasts)	3-5 days	6-12 months
All ground meat	1-2 days	3-4 months
Lunch Meats		
Prepackaged, unopened	2 weeks	
Opened	1 week	
Deli meats, sliced & handled	3-4 days	1 month
Seafood		
Raw lean fish		
(cod, flounder, sole)	1-4 days	6 months
Raw fatty fish (salmon, perch)	1-2 days	3 months
Raw shrimp	4 days	3 months
Cooked seafood	3 days	2 months
Dairy		
Uncooked eggs in shell	3 weeks	
Hard-cooked eggs in shell	1 week	6 months
Milk	5 days	1 month
Mayonnaise (opened)	2 months	

*QUICK TIP:
For information about meat and poultry safety in the United States, call the FDA at 202-720-2791.
For answers about seafood, call the FDA's hot line at 1-888-SAFE FOOD.
For general information, call 202-720-2791.

Sources:
-American Public Health Association
-United States Department of Agriculture
-Food and Drug Administration

❧ 4 ❧

The Balancing Protein Act
What is Protein?

Protein is an essential nutrient for life. It helps build new tissue, replaces damaged tissue, transports nutrients in and out of cells, regulates water and acid balance, transports oxygen and other nutrients that are found in the bloodstream, and is essential for making antibodies to help our immune systems fight disease and infection.

In The United States, the average citizen takes in far more protein than is needed to function optimally. In many countries, however, too few calories with too little protein (marasmus) or too little protein alone (kwashiorkor) are serious health problems that could prove fatal. Anyone who has seen a picture of a starving child who has stick-size arms and legs and a distended abdomen has seen severe protein-calorie depletion first-hand.

Too much or too little protein causes an imbalance in the body. Too little protein causes loss of energy, loss of nutrient balance, inability to grow normally, hair loss, constant food cravings, inability to heal, and a severely weakened immune system. Too much protein, especially from animal sources, has been implicated in heart disease, osteoporosis, obesity, and certain forms of cancer. Too much red meat, especially when consumed with calcium-rich foods, will cause calcium to be excreted in the urine, thus creating a potential risk for osteoporosis and electrolyte imbalance. In my counseling practice, I see more and more health-conscious individuals avoiding protein as though it were a dreaded disease. They wonder why they feel and look so awful and still can't lose weight. I continue to explain that if your body is lacking in essential nutrients, especially protein, your metabolism will slow down to conserve energy. Also, if dietary protein is too low, our bodies will utilize muscle for its protein source.

One of protein's most specific functions is to stimulate the production of the hormone glycogen. Glycogen's job is to open up the cells of stored fat already in the body for use as a fuel source. What this means is that eating protein in the form of poultry, fish, and red meat actually helps us lose weight by allowing our bodies to turn off the fat storage process so that we can begin burning fat for fuel.

HOW MUCH PROTEIN IS ENOUGH?

Our protein needs will differ, depending on age, sex, and activity level. For most adults, the portions recommended in Appendix A (Your Personal Food Plan) are ideal. For a safe protein intake for most adults, see also Table I on page 45 at the end of this chapter. A good rule of thumb for both children and adults is to **eat enough protein daily to equal the thickness and size of the palms of both hands.**

If you are totally vegan (consuming no animal foods or animal by-products), it is best to count **grams** instead of portions of protein because you can derive some protein from grains and high starch vegetables as well as from the obvious plant proteins such as nuts, seeds, and legumes (beans). If you consistently can't or won't consume enough food sources of protein, it is important to supplement with a protein concentrate, preferably from rice, soy, or egg whites.

PROTEIN FOR ATHLETES

Adequate protein intake is essential for all athletes. Protein boosts the metabolic rate and provides all the necessary amino acids to the body. It regulates the catabolic/anabolic cycle of the body, in which muscle tissue is broken down (catabolism) during strenuous physical activity and then rebuilt (anabolism). When protein is increased in the diet, the body forms new muscle. The higher your metabolic rate, the faster you are able to burn off fat stores and the better you utilize the energy foods you eat. In fact, an athlete who does not eat sufficient protein will not build muscle and/or lose fat efficiently.

How much and the best sources of protein for athletes during rigorous training should be assessed by a knowledgeable nutrition expert. The type of activity, age, target weight, number of calories burned, and target muscle building for the individual athlete need to be considered before an optimum protein intake can be recommended. It is also essential to keep in mind the best sources of protein (including protein powders) for the individual athlete are based on genetics, food sensitivities and/or food allergies. An optimum balance of protein with total carbohydrates and fats is also essential.

ARE HUMANS MEANT TO BE CARNIVORES?

According to Walter L. Voegtlin, M.D., in his book, *The Stone Age Diet*, Paleolithic man was a carnivore (animal eater) because we know a carnivore's gut-length is six times the animal's body length and is almost 100% efficient. The herbivore (plant eater) has a digestive tract 25 times the animal's body length and is only 50% efficient. It takes about 10,000 years to make functional and anatomical adaptations to an altered diet; thus, most humans today have had insufficient time to accomplish any but the most minor changes in the digestive tract. Since plant cellulose provides no nourishment for us, Dr. Voegtlin categorizes us as a carnivorous animal.

Voegtlin's assessment may not be entirely accurate for all humans today. First, although plant cellulose (fiber) cannot provide nourishment for humans, other nutrients from plants such as vitamins, minerals, carbohydrates and proteins are well utilized by humans. Secondly, the human small intestine varies by as much as 15 feet from person to person independent of sex, age, height, and weight. From my experience, genetics plays an important role in this phenomenon. The more ancient the DNA, as for most blood type O individuals, the shorter the small intestine appears to be. Blood type Os tend to thrive on generous portions of heavy red meats. Most blood type AB individuals, who typically have a more evolved DNA, tend to have longer intestinal tracts. Most AB's tolerate hard-to-digest plant foods, such as legumes, the best of any blood type. Genetic variation, therefore, still appears to play a major role in how much animal vs. vegetable protein is beneficial for humans in the 21st century (see Chapter 10 for an in depth discussion of genetic variation). The best classification for humans is OMNIVORE, defined as "animals intended to eat a wide variety of foods, both from animals and plants."

Paleolithic man, who lived from 1.6 million years ago to shortly before the advent of agriculture 10,000 years ago, ate far more animal protein than most humans do today. However, the wild game consumed by hunter-gatherers contained between 25-30% less fat than do today's domesticated animals. Not only is there more fat in domesticated animals, but the fat composition is different. Wild game has over five times as much unsaturated fat per gram when compared to high-in-saturated fat domesticated animals (*Science News*, Vol. 127, Feb. 9, 1985, p. 90) (S. B. Eaton, M. D., and M. Konner, Ph. D., "Paleolithic Nutrition," Vol. 312, *The New England Journal of Medicine*, No. 5, Jan. 31, 1985, pp. 283-289).

Even in the early 1900's, most beef in the United States was range-fed on large grasslands. A fatty acid called oleic acid naturally accumulated in the muscles of the cattle. Now, most beef cattle are fed grains and fattened up in feed lots with the help of the growth hormone stilbestrol. As a result, their muscles store up a different kind of fat, called stearic acid. Stearic acid promotes production of the bad LDL cholesterol, the one we want to keep low.

Most fowl (with the possible exception of chicken), do not appear to have been domesticated until several hundred years ago. The most commonly consumed fowl (now referred to as poultry) before that time were wild turkeys, quail, and other wild birds that were high in lean protein and low in saturated fat. They were also free of antibiotic and hormone residues that are so commonly used in animal feed in the United States today.

FREE-RANGE ANIMAL PROTEIN

Not only do free-range animals contain less body fat; but, until thirty years ago, almost all grazing animals that were used for food lived on grasses and other natural resources. They were not fed our modern domesticated animal diet of antibiotics, hormones, and pesticides nor were they fed ground meat and bone from other animals. Unfortunately, much of the animal food consumed in the United States today is contaminated with the residues of these dangerous substances. Thus, if you eat animal protein (red meat and fowl), it is imperative that you purchase only organic free-range varieties in U.S. markets and restaurants. Most of the European fowl and beef are already free of these substances. The good news is that organic free-range meats and poultry taste delicious!! Also, because of strict Jewish dietary laws and the way Kosher animals are slaughtered, Kosher animal foods are also presumably free of antibiotic, hormone, and pesticide residues.

HIGH CHOLESTEROL

The general assumption has been that high blood cholesterol levels are caused by high-cholesterol diets. In reality, many studies have not been able to prove any relation at all between cholesterol in the diet and serum cholesterol levels. One study, done on 4,000 people in Tecumseh, Michigan in 1976, determined only that there was a correlation between weight and cholesterol levels. The people who were overweight had high cholesterol levels, but their levels were not affected by eating foods high in dietary cholesterol.

The Framingham Heart Study, a famous ongoing study that has lasted for several decades, was designed to investigate the risk factors for heart disease. Although researchers did find that high (blood) serum cholesterol correlated strongly with heart disease, they were unable to prove any correlation between the consumption of high cholesterol foods such as eggs, fats, or meat with heart disease. Wanda Howell, an assistant professor of nutritional sciences at The University of Arizona, has been studying cholesterol for 28 years. She also concurs that dietary cholesterol has a minimal effect on serum cholesterol. However, she feels strongly that high serum cholesterol can be created by a diet high in saturated and hydrogenated fats. Also, diets lacking in essential fats and high in sugar and carbohydrates can increase serum cholesterol levels.

Keep in mind that some cholesterol is necessary in the diet; if we don't eat enough of it, our bodies actually accelerate cholesterol production. Cholesterol has some very vital functions in our bodies. That is why our cells manufacture it if it drops to a low level in our blood. Cholesterol is involved in the synthesis of sex hormones, protection of the myelin sheaths (the coating around nerves) in the brain, and in vitamin D and bile synthesis (involved in the digestion of fats). No matter what you eat, your cholesterol levels can actually increase under stress. Your body actually produces more cholesterol for the adrenal glands (our stress busters) to fight with much like the fight or flight reaction our ancestors needed to handle confrontations with wild animals.

FISH

Scientific research has shown fish to be an excellent source of protein, essential fatty acids (the Omega 3's) and minerals such as zinc, calcium, and magnesium. Most fish contain very little **saturated** fat. Of all the animal foods, fish is recommended most because of its tremendous health benefits. With regards to cancer, fish eaters are less likely to die of the disease than are non-fish eaters. A landmark research study, being performed by Dr. William Lane and approved of by the Food and Drug Administration is now testing shark cartilage for shrinking tumors and building human cartilage. Arthritic pain, stiffness, and swelling may be relieved by fish oil because of its anti-inflammatory properties. In fact, green-lipped mussels have been touted as an arthritic cure by many healers throughout the world. According to a recent Yale University study, eating only eight ounces of fish per week can cut the risk of having a heart attack by fifty percent! Salmon is one of the most perfect of all fish proteins because it is a rich source of calcium, magnesium, vitamin D, and the Omega 3 fatty acids, all of which contribute to excellent heart health and help prevent osteoporosis.

The Mediterranean Diet (which has now been endorsed by the European World Health Organization, the Harvard School of Public Health, and many prominent scientists) includes fish as one of the only recommended dietary sources of animal protein. Make sure that your fish comes only from deep ocean waters, rivers, seas, or clean lakes. Many lakes in the U.S., especially the Great Lakes, are not good sources for fish because the lakes have high levels of toxic agents, including PCB's and mercury. Farm-raised fish may be a problem if fed hormones or other "fattening agents." The larger the fish, the more toxic agents it will store.

Eggs are More than They're Cracked Up to Be

Eggs can be considered nature's perfect food because, if fertilized, they will grow into a living animal. Eggs have gotten a "bad rap" in the United States because they have been implicated in high serum cholesterol levels and heart disease. Although most eggs do contain a large amount of dietary cholesterol, there is no proof, according to the Framingham heart study, that moderate egg consumption (5–7 whole eggs per week) will cause high blood cholesterol levels. In fact, recent research has shown that egg consumption is clearly not a major cause of high blood cholesterol levels. It is, instead, the consumption of large amounts of saturated fats that are the leading culprits. An egg yolk contains only about 6 grams of total fat and only about 2 grams of that fat are saturated.

Gail Frank, professor of nutrition at California State University-Long Beach, calls an egg "the gold standard" of nutrition. An egg is an excellent source of protein (6-7 gms. per egg). The white is nature's highest quality of protein because it has a complete set of amino acids. An egg is easy to digest, which is especially helpful for young children and elderly adults. Also, the yolk, which cholesterol watchers often avoid like the plague, is an excellent source of lecithin (choline), B-12, and 11 other vitamins and minerals. Public opinion has scared off many elderly Americans from egg consumption. This is a shame because the egg is such an easy-to-chew, digestible, inexpensive form of protein.

Many egg manufacturers today have discovered that what they feed chickens affects the amount of cholesterol found in the chickens' eggs (isn't that a revelation?). So a diet lower in fat for the chicken will cause the eggs to be lower in cholesterol. Some egg manufacturers are even adding fish oil and flax to the chickens' diet so that the eggs will contain more vitamin E.

Ideally, you should eat, at most, only one yolk per day (but unrestricted whites) unless your cholesterol is extremely low. Be careful, however, to eat only organic eggs or eggs from free-range chickens. Otherwise, you'll be getting a large dose of pesticides, hormones, and antibiotic residues that not only make the eggs taste worse, but can also be damaging to your health. Also, you can make an egg high in fat, depending upon how you cook it. Continuously frying them in saturated fat and serving them with bacon on the side will definitely contribute to raised cholesterol levels.

Is Cow's Milk Really Nature's Perfect Food?

Dairy products, and cow's milk in particular, are not recommended sources of protein for most Americans. What animal in nature, after weaning, ever drinks the milk of another animal? Cow's milk is meant for calves. Cow's milk is not adaptable for most humans due to the tremendous difference in our digestive tracts and from an evolutionary standpoint. Milk as a food source for humans was introduced only about 10,000 years ago. Most adults who still have a functioning lactase enzyme after early childhood are descendants of people from dairying cultures. That is why anthropologists like Robert Dirks (professor of anthropology at Illinois State University and a specialist in food and culture) refers to cow's milk as an "ethnic" food.

In biblical times (beginning less than 10,000 years ago), humans consumed goat's and sheep's milk primarily. Even then, most adults consumed animal milk only after it was fermented into curds (for cheese) and yogurt to make it more digestible. Fermented milk products probably protected humans from harmful pathogens in biblical times as it does now because the fermentation process produced "friendly" intestinal flora to aid digestion and fight opportunistic pathogens such as yeast, salmonella, and shigella.

Cow's milk products, as produced in the United States today, bear no resemblance to milk consumed in most other countries and to raw milk as produced on organic farms (the most prevalent milk source in the U.S. until World War I). According to public health documents and many research studies, cow's milk is implicated in excess mucus production (related to sinus problems, asthma, ear and upper respiratory infections), digestive problems of intestinal gas, bloating, and diarrhea due to lactose intolerance (at least 75% of all adults are lactose intolerant) and severe constipation in children. The hormone and antibiotic adulteration of milk (see Chapter 3 for further details), the pesticides and other contaminants present in dairy cow's feed, and the chemical pasteurization and homogenization processes negate most of the nutritional benefits of cow's milk and make the fat, casein, and lactalbumin components of most milk products virtually impossible to digest.

When Washington D.C. based pediatrician, Russell Bunai, was asked what single change in the American diet would produce the greatest health benefit, he replied, "eliminating dairy products." We have been brainwashed by The U.S. Dairy Council to believe, first with The Four Food groups and now with the "Got Milk? advertising campaign, that cow's milk is the perfect food and that "you never outgrow your need for milk"). The scientific evidence against cow's milk as a human dietary staple grows yearly. Some of the most alarming studies follow.

Dr. Daniel Cramer, professor of obstetrics and gynecology and reproductive biology at Harvard Medical School, has researched a link between cow's milk consumption and ovarian cancer and infertility. He's not sure of the connection, but hypothesizes that it could involve the galactose (a metabolic by-product of milk sugar). Other speculation implicate the added estrogenic hormones given to the lactating cow that wind up in the milk that humans drink.

The American Academy of Pediatrics made a breast-feeding recommendation for the first year of a child's life due, in part, to research in the early 1990's implicating cow's milk and cow's milk based formulas with an increased risk for Type I diabetes in children. The research indicated the possibility of a genetic predisposition causing an autoimmune reaction to milk protein (casein).

Dr. Edward Giovannucci of Harvard Medical School and Harvard School of Public Health commented on emerging research findings and the results of his Health Professionals Study that implicate milk and excess calcium to a 4.5 greater risk of developing metastatic prostate cancer. Dr. Giovannucci feels that excess calcium, as found in milk, may shut down the body's production of Vitamin D, which protects the immune system.

Even the brainwashing of the American public which insists that milk consumption creates healthier bones (thus preventing Osteoporosis) research has never established this connection. In fact, the well-known Nurse's Health Study reported two years ago that older women who drank two or more glasses of milk per day had no greater protection from hip or forearm fractures than did women who drank one glass or less of milk per week. Absorbable calcium is the key to bone preservation, and for most of the human population, cow's milk is a poor choice.

For the sake of human health and disease prevention, it is best to avoid or minimize all cow's milk consumption, and then only from organic or imported sources. Occasional and small amounts of fermented dairy products, such as low fat cheese, kefir, and yogurt, are the best choices for adults. Milk from goats and sheep, especially if fermented, are probably the best daily choices for most humans.

So if We Don't Drink Milk, Where Will We Get Calcium?

High milk intake and better bones has not been established in any research, according to Dr. Meir Stampfer, Professor of Epidemiology and Nutrition at Harvard School of Public Health. To maintain proper calcium balance, it is essential to consume enough dietary calcium. Table II identifies optimum daily calcium intake for specific age groups, but contrary to the Dairy Council's assertion that we need to consume dairy products to get enough dietary calcium, excellent non-dairy and vegetarian sources of calcium are readily available and are listed in Table IV. Also, many fortified milk-substitute products have entered the American marketplace in direct response to the variety of problems associated with dairy products (see Table IV). Not only do these products, if fortified, provide similar nutrients to those found in milk, but they also may be used in cereals, baked goods, and other foods in which milk is typically added with no loss of mouth feel or flavor.

To prevent calcium loss, which contributes to degenerative diseases such as Osteoporosis, it is important to avoid overuse of phosphoric acid, found especially in soft drinks and red meat, and large amounts of both regular and decaffeinated coffee (over two cups daily for most people) or tea (over four cups daily for most people). The best absorption of calcium is found when it is accompanied by magnesium and Vitamin D. Tofu (and other soy products) and fish are natural sources of these nutrients. Could this be why small-boned oriental women, who eat their native diet, very rarely suffer from Osteoporosis?

Calcium also needs acid for optimum absorption. It is not wise for elderly people, who often are low in gastric acidity, to consume supplemental calcium in a carbonate form because calcium carbonate blocks stomach acid, thus preventing proper absorption of calcium. This lack of absorption may lead, in some cases, to bone and heel spurs, kidney stones, and calcification of the joints. The best absorption of supplemental calcium comes from calcium citrate, microcrystalline hydroxyapatite, or any form of calcium consumed with an acidic food, such as orange or grapefruit juice. For other factors affecting calcium absorption and optimum calcium sources, see Table III.

WHERE'S THE BEEF? NOT IN A VEGETARIAN DIET.

Too much animal protein, especially fatty cuts of meat, can cause a wide variety of health problems. Excess animal protein that cannot be utilized, will be excreted or stored as fat. On the other hand, a totally vegan diet (eating no animal food) may cause deficiencies of protein, dietary fat, vitamins, and minerals. Many individuals (especially blood type Os and Bs) cannot absorb and utilize a large amount of plant protein, but thrive on animal protein. To maintain good health, it is essential that your specific genetic needs be taken into consideration before you adopt a strict vegetarian diet.

According to studies of our paleolithic ancestors, the groups that consumed larger amounts of animal protein were larger boned and taller in stature than groups who could not find enough animal protein for food. With the advent of agriculture about 10,000 years ago, much more plant protein was consumed. The groups who consumed very little animal protein became smaller boned and smaller in stature. Today, the moderate protein intake of well-fed people living in the United States and Europe has created increases in height and bone size but not in body fat. Most people can tolerate a 25–75% plant protein diet. Variations of a vegetarian diet may include eggs, animal milk products, and fish. If genetically feasible, the following dietary recommendations should be considered for adults who choose to eat a vegan diet:

1. Consume at least two cups of cooked beans or four cups of soymilk and ½ cup of nuts/seeds or ¼ cup of nut or peanut butters (or any variation thereof) daily to meet protein needs.

2. For proper protein combining, because individual plant proteins are incomplete, consume at least one or two complementary grains daily. Ezekiel's Bread is an ideal biblical example of plant protein combining. Contrary to popular opinion, beans and grains do not have to be consumed together, but can be consumed at any time within a 24-hour period. Archaeologists and anthropologists have recently rediscovered a number of high protein grain-like foods, such as quinoa and amaranth, which may be used interchangeably with grains and legumes.

3. Take a supplement of B-12. In nature, B-12 is found only in animal foods. Supplement with extra zinc, calcium, magnesium, and iron if not enough can be derived from food. This would be particularly useful for pregnant/lactating women and athletes.

4. Avoid heavily processed and sugar laden foods completely to prevent depletion of B-vitamins, zinc, and magnesium.

LEGUMES

Legumes (beans), an excellent vegetarian food source, have been consumed by humans for over 10,000 years, according to expert nutritionist, Jean Carper, in her book entitled *Food – Your Miracle Medicine*. The ancient Greeks held "bean feasts" to honor the god, Apollo. The Egyptians put beans in the tombs of the Pharaohs as food to sustain them in the afterlife. There are also many biblical references identifying beans as a staple in their Mediterranean diet. In fact, much the sustenance supplied by Ezekiel's bread was derived from the perfect blend of a variety of beans, sprouted spelt, sprouted millet, and barley (see Chapter 5 for the Ezekiel's Bread recipe).

Beans are the healthiest, least perishable, and least expensive food for building good health. Beans can be counted as a protein or carbohydrate choice. Beans are high in fiber, vitamins, and minerals. They are also low in fat. Exciting research has shown that high blood cholesterol levels can drop by an average of 20 percent after several weeks of substituting beans for fatty meats. Beans also contain cancer-fighting compounds. But the best health news may be for hypoglycemics, diabetics, and dieters because beans stabilize blood sugar, thus triggering less hunger for high starch and high sugar foods.

There are a wide variety of legumes. The highest in protein is the soybean with its wonderful meat substitute or enhancement possibilities. Tofu, tempeh, and miso are often used instead of meat in hearty soups, stir-fries, pasta dishes, and stews. Soy yogurt, soymilk, and tofu are wonderful cow's milk substitutes. My personal soy snack favorites are edamame and soynuts. Other versatile legume varieties include adzuki, black, cannellini, fava, garbanzo (chickpeas), kidney, lentil, lima, navy, pinto, and white beans. String beans, peas, and peanuts are also classified as legumes.

Peanuts and peanut butter are a good source of plant protein. One-half cup of peanuts or one-fourth cup of peanut butter provides one serving of dietary protein. Peanuts are high in fat, but contain heart healthy monounsaturated fats. They are also good sources of B-6 and hard-to-get magnesium. Peanuts, in any form, should never be eaten raw or given to children under the age of two because they often contain an aflatoxin mold. This mold can be very toxic to an individual who has an underdeveloped immune system. Peanuts are the number one allergen of children living in the United States today, probably due to excess consumption too soon.

Many people have difficulty digesting beans due to weak enzyme function. Introducing them gradually to your diet may increase your tolerance. If not, adding a digestive enzyme such as bromelain (found naturally in fresh pineapple), papain (found naturally in papaya), or ginger when eating beans can help prevent flatulence and aid digestion.

NUTS ABOUT PROTEIN

Nuts and seeds are shunned by most weight-loss afficionados because they are high in fat. However, nuts and seeds, which have been around since Paleolithic times (see Chapter 10 for further details), get their fat from heart healthy monounsaturated fats. Nuts and seeds are also a powerhouse of hard-to-get vitamins and minerals such as vitamin E, B-complex, magnesium, calcium, and zinc. Recent research has proven that populations who consume large amounts of nuts and seeds are very heart healthy. In the last year, dietary recommendations for diabetics have included nuts, seeds, and beans because they all help stabilize blood sugar, which often decreases the diabetic's need for insulin.

Nuts and seeds are great for everyone, but are especially recommended for strict vegetarians, active children, rapidly growing teen-agers, endurance athletes, and pregnant women because they stabilize blood sugar, provide a good amount of necessary protein and fat, give energy, and assist in optimizing heart health. Eating one-fourth to one-half cup of raw nuts and seeds daily will ensure a beneficial amount without incurring unnecessary weight gain. For those individuals who have been told to avoid nuts and seeds because they suffer from diverticulitis or other digestive disorders, nut butters (such as almond butter, cashew butter, and sesame butter) are a delicious alternative.

PROTEIN IN A NUTSHELL

Protein is an essential nutrient; man cannot live for very long without it. Too little protein prevents growth or repair of damaged tissue. On the other hand, too much dietary protein, especially from red meat, is implicated in the promotion of degenerative diseases. Protein foods are abundant in nature and can provide good nutritional value from both animal and plant sources. Protein, consumed in moderation, is essential for optimum physical, mental, emotional, and spiritual health. Your personal choice of whether or not to eat strictly plant protein should bear in mind the fact that genetic heritage and ancestry, including blood type, are the keys as to what types of protein will build health and prevent disease.

Personal Case Study #4

Although I have seen hundreds of similar cases, Linda F.'s story stood out. She was a 37 year old full-time executive and mother of three young children who reported being "stressed out to the max." She had constant muscle pain, weight gain, trouble getting out of bed each morning and hair loss "by the buckets." Her doctor had told her that her problems were due to stress, but limiting her workload at home and on the job had made little difference.

Her food intake diary revealed almost all carbohydrates from bread products (bagels, toast, pretzels, etc.) and virtually no protein except for an occasional piece of skinless, boneless chicken breast or an egg white omelet. She also consumed too little fat.

I explained to her that her body was starving for protein and that her muscle pain was probably due to her body's survival mechanism of eating her muscle (bioavailable protein) for nourishment. Her metabolism had also slowed down to conserve energy due to her low protein intake, thus the weight gain and lack of energy. Lack of protein is also the second major cause of hair loss in women (the first is hormonal imbalance). Linda was reluctant to add more animal protein to her diet due to its inherent fat content, but was willing to try out our plan for one month.

When Linda had not returned several months later, I called her to ask how she was doing. She told me that she was too busy because she had been able to re-establish her old workload. She felt great, was almost back to her ideal weight and had regained her full head of hair. She said that even her children were "buying into" protein and healthy fats for brain function and athletic stamina.

TABLE I

PROTEIN SAFETY LEVELS FOR ADULTS

Adult Men	50–75 grams daily
Adult Women	45–65 grams daily
Pregnant/Lactating Women	75–90 grams daily

Sources:
USDA Dietary Guidelines
Staying Healthy with Nutrition, Elson M. Hass MD, 1999
Bowes & Church's Food Values of Portions Commonly Used,
     Jean A. Pennington, 1998

TABLE II

OPTIMUM CALCIUM INTAKE*

Infants		**Adults**	
Birth–6 months	360 mg.	Men	800 mg.
6 months–1 year	540 mg.	Women (18–24)	1200 mg.
		Women (25–50)	1000 mg.
		Pregnant Women	1200 mg.
Children		Lactating Women	1000 mg.
1–10 years	800 mg.	Post-menopausal	1200 mg.
11–18 years	1,000 mg.	Women	1500 mg.

Sources:
–(United States Dept. of Health and Human Services, 1998
–(Institute of Medicine, Food and Nutrition Board. Dietary reference intakes for calcium phosphorus mg., Vitamin D and Fluoride. Washington D.C., National Academy Press 1997.
* 500–800 mg. daily calcium intake may be acceptable for most adults if losses are minimal, an equal amount of magnesium and at least 400 i.u. of vitamin D are consumed concurrently, and the sources of calcium are optimally absorbed.

TABLE III

CALCIUM ABSORPTION

Factors Affecting Calcium Absorption

Increased By:
- Body needs – growth, pregnancy, lactation
- Vitamin D
- Magnesium
- Acid environment – hydrochloric acid, citric acid, ascorbic acid (vitamin C)
- Exercise

Decreased By:
- Vitamin D deficiency
- Magnesium deficiency
- Gastrointestinal problems
- Hypochlorhydria (low stomach acid)
- Stress
- Lack of exercise
- Calcium carbonate (turns off stomach acid)
- High fat intake
- High animal protein intake
- Excess coffee & tea
- High phosphorus intake
- Oxalic acid foods (beet greens, chard, spinach, rhubarb, cocoa)
- Phytic acid foods (whole wheat)

Types of Calcium Supplements: Their Advantages and Disadvantages

Types	Advantages	Disadvantages
Microcrystalline Hydroxyapatite Concentrate (25% calcium)	• very well absorbed calcium source • complete bone food • can reduce bone loss • absorbed by many malabsorbers	NONE
Citrate (24% calcium)	• very well absorbed • reduced risk of kidney to kidney stones • absorbed by those with poor digestion	• not a complete bone food
Aspartate (20% calcium)	• well absorbed	• not a complete bone food
Amino Acid Chelate (10-20% calcium)	• well absorbed	• not a complete bone food • may irritate MSG/Nutrasweet® or soy sensitivities
Ascorbate (10% calcium)	• well absorbed • non acidic vitamin C	• not a complete bone food
Lactate (15% calcium)	• well absorbed	• not a complete bone food • may contain milk or yeast by-products • made from fermentation of molasses whey, starch, sugar with calcium carbonate

Types of Calcium Supplements: Their Advantages and Disadvantages *(continued)*

Types	Advantages	Disadvantages
Carbonate (40 % calcium)	• cheapest source of calcium (Tums®) with poor stomach digestion	• not a complete bone food • may be malabsorbed by those • antacid effect, interferes with digestion/absorption & causes gas and constipation
Bone Meal (39% calcium)	• contains multiple minerals needed for bone	• may contain high lead,arsenic, cadmium, etc.

Sources:
The Calcium Bible by Patricia Hausman.
Metagenics, Inc.
Staying Healthy with Nutrition by Elson Haas, M.D.

TABLE IV
CALCIUM CONTENT OF FOODS*
(Non-dairy Choices)

Food Item	Calcium (mg.)	Food Item	Calcium (mg.)
Almonds (1/2 cup)	160	Parsley (1 cup)	80
Blackberries (1/2 cup)	45	Peanuts (1/2 cup)	110
Bok Choy (1 cup)	250	Pecans (1/2 cup)	40
Broccoli (1 cup)	40	Salmon, canned pink (4 oz.)	220
Brussel sprouts (1 cup)	50	Salmon, canned red (4 oz.)	290
Cabbage (1 cup)	35	Sardines, canned with bones	
Carrots (1 cup)	45	(4 oz.)	500
Celery pieces (1 cup)	40	Scallops, fresh (4 oz.)	130
Collard Greens (1 cup)	290	Seaweed, hijiki (1/2 cup)	300
Corn tortilla, lime-treated (3.5 oz.)	300	Shrimp, fresh (4 oz.)	130
Dandelion greens (1 cup)	205	Soybeans, cooked (1 cup)	140
Haddock (3 oz.)	210	Spinach, raw (1 cup)	200
Kale (1 cup)	150	Squash, cooked (1 cup)	55
Kidney beans (1 cup)	75	Sunflower seeds, raw (1/2 cup)	65
Lima beans (1 cup)	65	Sweet potatoes, cooked (1 cup)	50
Milk substitutes (1 cup)**	200–300	Tilapia, fresh farm-raised (4 oz.)	120
Mackerel, canned (4 oz.)	300	Tofu (4 oz.)	145
Mustard greens (1 cup)	60	Tofu, enriched (4 oz.)	280
Tuna, oil-packed (3 oz.)	200	Turnip greens (1 cup)	250
Navy beans (1 cup)	100	Walnuts (1/2 cup)	50
Orange (1 medium)	55	Watercress (1 cup)	40
Orange juice (calcium fortified)	300		

*The amounts of calcium listed above are approximations; organically grown items may contain more calcium and overly processed foods may contain less.
**For a list of milk substitutes, see "Non-Dairy Milk Substitutes."

Source: *Bowes & Church's Food Values of Portions Commonly Used*, Jean A.
Pennington, 1998

NON-DAIRY MILK SUBSTITUTES

Product	Description	Nutritional Information
Rice Milk Pacific Rice Drink (fat free) Pacific Rice Lowfat Rice Dream (enriched) Westbrae Rice Beverage	organic rice milk in flavors such as original, vanilla, carob, and chocolate; great for people who have soy allergies, gluten intolerance, or digestive problems; the taste is pleasant; children often prefer the chocolate flavor	low in fat; no saturated fat; very digestible for most people; enriched to match or surpass cow's milk fortification; 20–30% daily calcium requirement
Soy Milk Pacific Soy Fat-Free ProSoya "So Nice" Soydream West Soy Plus West Soy Nonfat White Wave Silk Edensoy	made from soybeans (see benefits of legumes); contains some protein; has a perfect balance of calcium and magnesium; the fortified soy milk is great for toddlers who are weaning from soy formula	1–5 fat grams; 90–100 calories per serving; no cholesterol; enriched to match or surpass cow's milk fortification; 20–30% daily calcium requirements; 2–6 grams of protein

✠ 5 ✠

Cut the "Carbos"
Too Much of a Good Thing

There is a misconception in the United States, especially promoted by the USDA Food Pyramid, that we can maintain or lose weight by avoiding fats and limiting proteins. But when we cut back on the foods that give us a full feeling and stabilize blood sugar, our natural tendency is to eat more carbohydrates to satisfy hunger. Consuming large amounts of carbohydrates will cause weight gain. This is why if you consume the Food Pyramid's daily recommended carbohydrate choices of 6–11 grains, 3–5 vegetables (with no differentiation between high and low starch), 2–4 fruits, and minimally added sugar you probably will gain weight. Since the USDA Food Pyramid has been used as a guideline for optimum food portions, Americans have become more overweight today than at any other time in history! USDA recommendations allow for too many carbohydrates for most people to consume in a day. In this chapter we will identify all high starch foods as carbohydrates and explain their benefits and risks in detail.

BREAD—THE STAFF OF LIFE

Whole grains (from which bread originated) have played an important role in the lives of human beings since they first learned that planting and harvesting foods could provide them with a constant supply of nourishment so that they could give up their nomadic ways. Bread baking began in ancient Egypt as early as 4000 B.C., and ancient bread was typically made from wheat, barley, and spelt. There are more biblical references to bread and grains than to any other food group. In fact, in the book of

Ezekiel, it was said that a man "could live for 1 year with no more than a specified portion of this bread recipe and water" (see recipe for Ezekiel's Bread on page 51). Commercial versions of Ezekiel's bread are available today (see "Natural Foods Shopping Tour" in Appendix B). The reason ancient breads are so healthful and digestible is because they are sprouted. The "sprouting" allows for their powerful enzymes to digest the carbohydrates and fiber in the bread.

Unfortunately, most whole wheat bread made commercially today bears little resemblance to ancient bread and is very hard to digest. Also, because whole wheat is an insoluble fiber, it aids in elimination but may block essential mineral absorption. For my clients with irritable bowel syndrome, Crohn's, or any digestive problem, we eliminate all wheat for at least two weeks. If my clients feel better when not eating wheat and worse when adding it back, we will recommend that they avoid it completely for three to six months; then rotate it on a five day basis if they can tolerate it occasionally.

Breads that include grains other than whole wheat are more digestible for most people and cause less weight gain. These include rice, rye, oat, and millet breads. The white, light, spongy, and smooth "bread" that has been stripped of its food value is not recommended. Chemicals, including bleach, are often added to make bread look pure white. When any grain is highly refined by overprocessing, the outer layer (the fiber-containing bran layer) is removed. The inner embryo or germ, wherein lie the greatest concentration of nutrients, is also removed. The refined flour that remains has, thus, undergone a tremendous loss of nutrients. It is virtually impossible to lose or maintain weight when eating large amounts of overprocessed or heavily refined bread. The ideal portion of bread for anyone watching their weight is 1–2 slices daily maximum. For my clients who want to lose weight, we eliminate ALL bread for one month, then rotate multi-grain or sprouted whole wheat bread not more than once every 4 days until they have reached their ideal weight.

Ezekiel's Bread

Nutritionists have discovered that bread made from a variety of grains delivers more food value and higher quality protein than breads made from a single grain. This is called the principle of augmentation, according to Reuben Hubbard and Don Hawley, who are nutritionists and authors of *Health Secrets of the Bible* (Loma Linda University School of Health, 1979).

Ezekiel's Bread will supply all the essential nutrients including protein, fat, calcium, phosphorous, iron, sodium, potassium, Vitamins A and C, magnesium, zinc, thiamine, riboflavin, and niacin. Plus, it tastes great! The equivalent of one cup of this dough made into bread and eaten daily would allow a human to survive for at least a year, if the sixth part of a hin (approximately 3 cups) of water is also consumed daily.

Recipe for Ezekiel's Bread:

8 cups of sprouted wheat

2 cups sprouted soy beans

¼ cup sprouted spelt

½ cup warm water

4–5 T. extra virgin olive oil

2 packets yeast in ½ cup warm water

malted barley (keep adding for proper consistency)

4 cups sprouted barley

½ cup sprouted millet

1 cup sprouted lentils

1 T. sea salt

1 T. raw honey

½ cup organic all-purpose whole grain flour (keep adding for proper consistency)

Dissolve the yeast in the water and let it sit for 10 minutes. Pulverize sprouted ingredients in a blender. Mix in all with the remaining ingredients. Add the yeast mixture last. Knead the dough with with a small amount of all-purpose flour (so that the mixture won't stick) until smooth. Put into an oiled bowl and cover the bowl with a towel. Let the dough rise until double in bulk. Knead the dough again. Cut the dough and shape into loaves. Place the dough into greased pans. Let the dough rise again. Bake at 375 degrees for 45 minute to one hour. Yield: 4 small loaves

Grains

Grains have been food staples and the main source of nourishment for most of the world's countries for thousands of years. Wheat is a staple food for over half of the world. More wheat is eaten than any other grain in the world today and provides half of the dietary calories for 1.6 billion people. Rice is the second most consumed grain worldwide and is a food staple of China, Japan, and Africa, is very high in B-vitamins, and is one of the least allergenic grains. Barley is presently a staple of Tibet, China, and Japan. Barley is wonderful for digestion and prevention of constipation. It also contains a healthy amount of protein, helps to lower blood cholesterol levels, and is an important grain of the brewing industry. Corn is the least complete grain nutritionally, but contains large amounts of fiber. Corn, in the form of maize (Indian corn), was worshipped by many Native Americans throughout history. Because it is cheap to grow and process, corn is the most commonly used grain in the U.S., but also is one of the most common allergens. Grains such as rye, millet, oats, spelt, and sorghum are consumed worldwide, but to a lesser extent than wheat, rice, and corn. Ancient grainlike foods, such as quinoa and amaranth, are regaining popularity in whole foods markets today due to their nutritional superiority and less allergenic potential. If refined grains are enriched to make up for some of the vitamins and minerals and are free of chemicals, they also can be well worth eating. (See pages 155–158 of the Natural Organic Foods List for specific brands.)

The USDA Food Pyramid encourages the popular belief that whole grains are a highly beneficial food for Americans. Except for ancient wild grasses (see Chapter 10 for further details), most grains are incompatible with about 60% of the world's population. For most of the world's population, where starvation or survival are the key issues, grains are an inexpensive, readily available source of nourishment. But in the United States where overnutrition, obesity, and blood sugar imbalances (especially in the forms of hypoglycemia and diabetes) are escalating, excess grain consumption is not recommended. Most grains (both refined and unrefined) are high on the glycemic index, and thus will release too much insulin. With each dose of grain, especially if not balanced with protein or fat, excess insulin will be secreted, insulin levels will rise and fall too quickly, and a false hunger signal will be released by the brain, causing more hunger cravings. A vicious cycle of carbohydrate craving has become the norm in many American households.

Too many carbohydrates are not only implicated in poor blood sugar regulation, but a recent study in the American Journal of Cardiology (*Am J of Cardiol 2000*, 85: 45–48) reported that a high carbohydrate diet elevates triglycerides and lowers HDL (good) cholesterol. Thus, a high carbohydrate diet can now be considered a causative factor for heart disease.

My recommendation for eating grains is to choose a wide variety of compatible, non-allergenic whole grains in limited amounts (maximum of two servings daily for most Americans) and always eat them accompanied by some protein or fat for proper insulin balance.

A cup of cooked whole grains contains, on average, 200 calories and is easy to prepare. Whole grains are rich in complex carbohydrates, B-vitamins, and contain traces of the minerals magnesium, calcium, iron, and zinc. A cup of grain can offer anywhere from 3 grams of fiber (millet) to 5 grams (corn grits) to as much as 10 or 11 grams (oats, rye, whole wheat, or buckwheat). Grains are versatile: you can eat them hot at breakfast or serve them with a meal as a balance to your choice of protein.

Following is a list of basic grains and grain-like foods. Many are sold in supermarkets; the more exotic ones are found primarily in specialty shops or health-food stores. Because of their high oil content, whole grains spoil quickly and need to be kept in the refrigerator or freezer.

Amaranth. SEE "Quinoa".

Arrowroot. A tropical American plant with starchy roots. The thickening agent, arrowroot powder, comes from the root of this plant. It blends well with most flours and because it is so airy, brings out the flavors of whatever it thickens (such as stir-fry). It is completely safe for gluten-free diets.

Barley. Available as "pot" or "Scotch" barley (whole kernels) or as "pearl" (polished), this glutenous grain is versatile. It is great in soups, stews, for side dishes, and as a breakfast cereal. It is also used to brew beer and whiskey. Because sprouted barley is high in the sugar, maltose, barley malt is used to sweeten a wide variety of packaged foods. Like oats, barley may lower blood cholesterol. Barley tea and water are often used to soothe colicky babies and people suffering from flatulence and indigestion.

Buckwheat. The groats are not a true grain, but a seed from the thistle plant in the rhubarb family. Roasted and ground buckwheat is called kasha, which can be cooked like rice for a side dish. Buckwheat flour can be mixed with wheat to make bread and pancakes. Buckwheat's nutty flavor makes it a good food choice for people with grass and/or grain allergies, but should be avoided by individuals on gluten-free diets.

Corn. Though a true grain, corn takes many forms such as corn-on-the-cob, hominy (hull and germ removed and usually used as a side dish), grits (dried hominy used for cereal and side dishes), polenta (coarse-ground Italian cornmeal used like a bread as an accompaniment to many side dishes), and masa harina (a specially prepared cornmeal for tortillas). Corn comes in many colors: red, blue (used mostly for corn chips and popcorn), yellow, and white (used more in bread and muffin baking). Corn contains no gluten. Corn is a staple in the U.S. It is concentrated into a powder or syrup to sweeten processed foods and used as thickener and starch in many vitamin/mineral pills as well as in medications. Corn is also a commercial source of fructose, dextrose, xylitol and sorbitol. Is it any wonder that corn has become one of the most common allergens in the U.S.?

Flax. Although listed botanically as a seed, this high fiber food has been added to bread and cakes for thousands of years. Preliminary scientific research has shown flax to speed up the transit time in the digestive tract and to be a valuable preventive for colon cancer. Flax is high in Omega 3 essential fatty acids (see Chapter #6 for benefits). It is also recommended in the treatment of female disorders and promotes healthy nails, bones, teeth, and skin.

Job's Tears. These ripe seeds of a tall grass are so ancient that they still bear their original biblical name. Job's Tears are a heritage grain of China and Japan. This non-gluten grain has a wonderful nutty flavor.

Kamut. Triticum polinicum, nicknamed King Tut's wheat, is a large kerneled pasta wheat. Because it is a cousin of wheat, it is not recommended on a wheat or gluten-free diet.

Millet. High in phosphorus and B vitamins, millet is used chiefly as animal feed in the U.S., but makes a nutritious side dish, cereal, or flavor enhancer in bread. Early research indicates that millet does contain gluten, but not as much as wheat or rye.

Oats. A glutenous grain that is sold in many forms. Whole kernels (groats) must cook for an hour. Irish or steel-cut oats take about 40 minutes and make a wonderful, chewy breakfast. Flattened rolled oats take only minutes and are delicious but softer. Oatmeal processed into flour in a blender can be used in breads, muffins, and pancakes. Oats may lower blood cholesterol; and because they are a soluble fiber, help digestion and elimination without causing bloating.

Quinoa and Amaranth. Amaranth and Quinoa are called "Supergrains" because they were energizing food staples of the Aztec, Mayan and Central American Indians. They can be a good substitute for people with grass/grain allergies. They may be cooked whole and ground into flour from the whole grain. Amaranth and quinoa are high in protein, fiber, and amino acids (unlike most grains, they contain lysine and methionine). Three tablespoons of these flours have more protein and calcium than one-half cup of milk. They are often grown organically. Quinoa is not sticky like some high gluten grains because it is virtually gluten free. It is light, tasty, and easy to digest. Amaranth has a stronger, nutty flavor. You may want to use an additional type of flour and spices when baking with amaranth if it seems too pungent.

Rice. The second most consumed grain in the world, rice is a staple food throughout much of Asia. It is also popular in the U.S. due to its mild taste, versatility, digestibility, and few allergic reactions. If not polished to remove the fiber or highly refined, it is a major source of B-vitamins. It is also gluten-free.

Rye. Its low gluten content produces dense bread, so rye is usually mixed with other grains when used in bread baking. Whole rye kernels, known as rye berries, are sold in health-food stores and may be used like whole-wheat berries for side dishes or salads.

Sorghum. Historically referred to as Syrian grass, is the third most consumed grain in the world. It is grown primarily in Africa, China, India, and the U.S. It has a nuttier flavor than wheat and is often used to feed cattle, as a cereal, and to sweeten foods. Sorghum is gluten-free.

Spelt. A staple of West Germany and a cousin to wheat, spelt has a slightly stronger flavor but maintains a good amount of gluten and elasticity. This makes it excellent for baking breads, muffins, and cakes. Because it contains gluten and is closely associated with wheat, spelt is not recommended for those suffering from gluten intolerance or wheat allergies.

Tapioca. Comes from the starchy root of the tropical plant, cassava. It is excellent as a thickener for soups and gravies. It can also be finely ground into a flour consistency so it can be used in bread or pudding. It is almost universally non-allergenic, well-digested, and gluten-free.

Tef (or tef grass).   Commonly found in health food stores; it has a high nutrient density. It can, however, cause allergic reactions to those individuals suffering from grass/grain allergies and is not recommended for a gluten-free diet.

Triticale.   A hybrid of wheat and rye. It is popular in Scandinavia. Triticale has a high protein content with a good balance of amino acids. It is high in gluten.

Wheat.   This is the oldest and most highly consumed grain in the world. Its sweet, nutty flavor and wide varieties make it very versatile. It comes in the form of whole or cracked berries. Bulgur (crushed parboiled wheat) is used to make tabouli. Durum (Semolina) is a hard mold-resistant winter wheat that is great for making pasta and can be ground into flour to make a chewy, high protein bread. Flour made from soft wheat is good for making bread, pancakes, and baked goods. It is a favorite of bakers due to its high elasticity and gluten content. Couscous is a variety of semolina that is commonly consumed in the Middle East and was discovered over 4,000 years ago. It tastes very similar to pasta (although the kernel size is about the same size as rice) and is great as a balanced protein combined with beans. Wheat is a very common allergen.

Wild Rice.   In its pure form (Oryza fatua or O. spontanea) it is not really rice; it is a wild grass. Because it has a nutty, almost musty flavor, it is a great accompaniment for game meats and fowl. It is also appropriate for a gluten-free diet. Wild rice is very expensive so it is often mixed into a rice pilaf by adding other forms of rice.

GRAIN ALLERGIES

Millions of individuals, world-wide, are intolerant of one or more grains due to food allergy, gluten intolerance, or lack of digestive enzymes needed to digest grains. The occurrence of allergenic reactions to the most commonly consumed grains are reported as follows:

Most Likely to be Allergenic	Less Likely	Least Likely
Corn	Barley	Amaranth
Rye	Buckwheat	Arrowroot
Triticale	Flax	Quinoa
Wheat	Job's Tears	Rice
	Kamut	Tapioca
	Millet	Wild Rice
	Oats	
	Sorghum	
	Spelt	
	Tef	

For people with one or more grain allergies, substitutions can easily be made using other grains, grain-like foods, or high starch vegetables to make delicious breads, pancakes, and baked goods. Many of these substitutes are gluten-free, which are beneficial for those individuals who are gluten intolerant, including those suffering from celiac or sprue. Some of these are highlighted as follows:

GRAIN AND HIGH STARCH VEGETABLE SUBSTITUTIONS FOR ONE CUP OF ALL-PURPOSE WHEAT FLOUR:

- ½ cup arrowroot or tapioca with ½ cup of ground nut meal (grain allergy, gluten intolerance)
- 7/8 cup buckwheat, quinoa or amaranth flour (grain allergy)
- ¾ cup cornstarch or 7/8 cup corn flour (gluten intolerance)
- 5/8 cup potato flour or ¾ cup potato starch (gluten intolerance, grain allergy, easy to digest)
- ¾ cup oat flour or 1½ cups rolled oats, ground (wheat allergy)
- ¾ cup rice flour with 1 tsp. baking soda (gluten intolerance, most grain allergies, easy to digest)
- ¾ cup soy, barley, millet, or bean flours* with 1 tsp. baking soda

*Bean Flours—Flours can be made from any starchy veg-
etable, legume or grain. Legume (bean) flours are very
hard, which makes them difficult to grind. Use a coffee or
seed grinder for best results. Process according to manu-
facturer's directions. Process into a fine powder. Try soak-
ing beans overnight in water, then finely grind into a
"mush." Decrease the amount of liquid used in the recipe
to compensate for the water that has been soaked into
the beans.

High Starch Vegetables

High starch vegetables are included in the Carbohydrate
section of your Personal Food Plan because they are a
valuable source of easy-to-digest starch, give a feeling of
fullness like grains, and are a good choice as a grain sub-
stitution for those suffering from grain allergies, digestive
difficulties, or gluten intolerance. They may, however,
cause weight gain if eaten in excess. English (white) potatoes, sweet potatoes, yams, English peas, beans (legumes),
corn (kernel or on-the-cob), and carrots are examples of
high starch vegetables. People who regularly snack on
baby carrots may satisfy their sweet tooth, but may notice
extreme blood sugar swings if they are eaten alone due to
having a high glycemic index count (about 92%).

The vitamin and mineral content of most high starch
vegetables is very high, and scientific research is uncover-
ing new information about their health benefits every
day. For instance, sweet potatoes have been found to contain a large amount of beta carotene, a cancer preventive
and powerful antioxidant. Beta carotene, as a precursor to
Vitamin A, is non-toxic in foods, even in large amounts.
Wild yams have been found to sometimes provide unbe-
lievable relief for women suffering from hormonal imbalances, including Premenstrual Syndrome and Menopause.
Wild yam cream is even being touted today for the prevention of Osteoporosis.

Legumes, in particular, have shown benefits as an
excellent source of fiber, bringing down total and LDL

blood cholesterol levels, assisting in blood sugar and blood pressure regulation, and more recently as a powerful cancer preventative. Soybeans, fermented forms such as miso, tofu, and tempeh, contain phytoestrogens to regulate menopausal symptoms and replace harmful xenoestrogens (cancer-causing agents) in estrogen receptor sites. The U.S. Food and Drug Administration has now authorized heart health claims for soy, which state, "25 grams of soy protein a day, as part of a diet low in saturated fat and cholesterol, may reduce the risk of heart disease." Soy also has a plentiful amount of protein (see Chapter #4), so it is an excellent source of nourishment for vegetarians.

FRUIT

Grapes and figs were two of the most frequently consumed foods during biblical times. Today we know that they are high in antioxidants that prevent disease-causing free radical formation. Figs, even as far back as 2,000 years ago, were used by the Israelite king, Hezekiah, to cure his presumably cancerous growth. For centuries, figs have also have been recommended for treatment of cancer, constipation, scurvy, hemorrhoids, gangrene, liver conditions, skin eruptions like boils, and low energy. Science has caught up with folklore because an active agent in figs, called benzaldehyde, has been used successfully in advanced cancers of both mice and humans. An enzyme in figs, called ficin, has also been shown to aid digestion.

Grapes are only second to apples as the queen of fruits. Although grapes have benefited human health for centuries, it has taken until the late twentieth century for them to earn a place in scientific research. We now know that the polyphenols and tannins found in grapes are powerful antiviral and antitumor agents. To receive all benefit and no risk from the active ingredients in grapes, they should always be organically grown.

Prunes, a dried fruit similar to figs in taste and mouth feel, are commonly believed to be nothing more than a laxative to promote regularity. But thanks to research, prune puree is now being used commercially in low-fat baking to replace the fat from butter or margarine. Prune puree retains the moisture in baked goods, requires less sweeteners and tastes delicious while still aiding elimination.

Almost every fruit and vegetable can tell its own story of health-building and disease fighting. Some of the greatest benefits have been seen with concentrated extracts and juicing. Delicious, freshly squeezed juices are a great alternative to soft drinks and alcohol and may be enjoyed by young and old alike. Table III highlights delicious and nutritious juice recipes adapted from Michael T. Murray's book, *A Complete Book of Juicing.*

WINE—THE FRUIT OF THE VINE

Wine is one of the few alcoholic beverages that, in moderation, shows tremendous health benefits. A 5-ounce glass of wine may be counted as one serving of carbohydrates. Wine was a staple in ancient times for several reasons, but especially because water was either scarce or polluted and wine would not rot quickly. The benefits of moderate wine-drinking have recently been tested scientifically. Small amounts of wine, especially red wine, can prevent plaque from growing in arteries to the heart; can raise the "good" HDL blood cholesterol, can assist in killing bacteria and viruses, and aids in digestion of large meals by stimulating the production of gastric juice. Some of the healthiest populations of the world are wine-drinking cultures. In the United States, organic wines that are certified sulfite-free are the safest.

SIMPLE SUGARS

Humans have "craved" sugar from the beginning of time. Nature intended for man to enjoy the taste of sweet foods because that was the best way for ancient man to know if a food was ripe (fruits and vegetables become sweeter as they ripen) and was an accurate way of testing the safety of plant foods. Poisonous plants usually are bitter; thus, ancient man would have wanted to avoid them except in times of famine. Plants essential for nutritional value often tasted sweet so that ancient man would be encouraged to eat them.

Biblical passages refer to natural sweets often, in terms of delicacies or gifts. Because "sweets" were delicacies or gifts, they would not have been consumed in large quantities. Raw, uncooked honey was considered a "sweet" delicacy and has been around since early Paleolithic times. Raw honey, available in most health food and grocery stores today, is very nutrient dense, if consumed in small portions. Honey should not be consumed by children under the age of two.

REFINED VS. NATURAL SUGARS

Sugar is the smallest unit of carbohydrate produced by a plant. There are many different kinds of sugar, depending upon their chemical structures. Sugar is referred to as a "simple carbohydrate" because its molecular chains are much shorter than are the molecular chains of complex carbohydrates. Naturally occurring sugars are found within many plant foods and in the milk of most mammals. When naturally occurring sugars (i.e. sugar cane, beets, corn, lactose from milk, honey from bees, etc.) are over-processed and chemically altered, the resultant compound is referred to as a refined sugar, which is stripped of nutrients and metabolized poorly by the body. Some of the most common refined sugars are referred to on food labels as sucrose, lactose, fructose, corn sugar, cane sugar, sorbitol, glucose, maltose, dextrose, corn sweetener, beet sugar, and brown sugar.

Table I identifies both natural and refined sugars and lists their nutritional values. From the nutrient levels listed, it is easy to see that processing of natural sugar depletes food value.

Most refined sugars are referred to as empty calories, because they provide no nutritional value along with their calories. The average American consumes 600 "empty" calories each day. If you're on a weight loss diet, this could be providing half of your daily caloric intake! It's not always easy to avoid refined sugar because many packaged foods contain hidden sugars that consumers may not even be aware they're eating. For instance, did you know that most commercially prepared catsup derives 33% of its calories from added sugar? Yet, catsup may still be classified as a **vegetable** by the U.S. Department of Agriculture.

Besides providing "empty calories," refined sugars are often eaten to excess. It is not easy to eat naturally occurring sugars to excess because they are filling, especially dried fruits. How many of us, for instance, could eat a whole box of prunes in one sitting? With refined sugar, however, a few tablespoons give us the "sugar" equivalent of an entire box of prunes, as well as a host of chemicals such as chlorine bleach and formaldehyde that our bodies have to attempt to detoxify. Eating excess sugar often causes sugar addiction because more than about two teaspoons of sugar (the equivalent of 4 ounces of most soft drinks) consumed without nutrient dense foods will cause the pancreas to oversecrete insulin, resulting in a drop in blood glucose and the depletion of valuable vitamins and minerals. The way most of us treat the symptoms of low blood glucose levels is by eating more sugar. Thus, we set the stage for riding a roller coaster of physical, mental, and emotional highs and lows. This problem is worse for most children naturally than for adults because children have more erratic blood glucose levels. The average American consumes about 130 pounds of refined sugar each year! Excess refined sugar consumption contributes to many health problems, including dental cavities, obesity, high blood triglycerides and cholesterol levels (when combined with saturated fat), a weakened immune system, pancreatic exhaustion, and a depletion of vitamins and minerals.

Sugars should be consumed in moderation because their carbohydrate content is very concentrated. One tablespoon of simple sugar is the equivalent of about one cup of high starch vegetables or ¾ cup of cooked grain.

SUGAR SUBSTITUTES

Sugar substitutes are often thought to be a panacea for the insatiable human sweet tooth. Three of the most common sugar substitutes consumed in the U.S. have been cyclamate, saccharin, and Aspartame (Nutrasweet®). There have been problems associated with these three "sweet fixes." Several others, Acesulfam-K, Stevia, and Sucralose, have so far shown no serious adverse reactions.

Properties of the most common sugar substitutes are as follows:

Cyclamate. This has been around the longest. A ban was imposed on it in the U.S. in 1970 after it was found to cause cancer in laboratory animals. Cyclamate is 30 times sweeter than sugar and has no calories.

Saccharin. Contains no calories and is about 300 times sweeter than sugar. Since 1977, the U.S. Food and Drug Administration has threatened a ban because of evidence linking it to bladder cancer in animals. Warning labels now advise consumers of those findings.

Aspartame. (Nutrasweet®) For a short time seemed to be the perfect sugar substitute. It's derived from two amino acids (aspartic acid and phenylalanine) so it is touted as being natural. It is also 200 times sweeter than sugar and has tremendous taste appeal. But, alas, all is not paradise. The longer it has been used, the more problems researchers and consumers have uncovered. It has been found to be an excitotoxin to the brain, which means that it overstimulates and kills brain cells. The Centers for Disease Control in the United States have reported over 6,000 side effects from Nutrasweet®, including blurred vision, permanent blindness, seizures, and even death. For a detailed discussion of Nutrasweet®, see Chapter #2.

Acesulfam-K. (Sunette®, Sweet One®) A synthetic odorless white crystal that has reported no major complications, probably because its uses have been limited. Center for Science in the Public Interest has voiced suspicions that Acesulfam-K may be carcinogenic and that studies were poorly done.

Stevia. (see page 49 for "Natural Ways to Satisfy your Sweet Tooth")

Sucralose. Approved by the FDA in 1998. It is the only sweetener that is made from sugar, tastes like sugar, and can be used anyway sugar would be used. Sucralose is the most thoroughly safety tested food additive in the world. Since millions of consumers have used this product since 1991 with no major side effects, it appears safe.

Unfortunately, most sugar substitutes have not contributed to weight loss as hoped. In fact, Dr. Walter Willet, a Harvard University Nutrition expert, reported studies that showed the highest common denominator for women who **gained** weight was the use of artificial sweeteners. Also, products containing sugar substitutes usually have no nutritional value (i.e. gum, candy, soft drinks, desserts).

NATURAL WAYS TO SATISFY YOUR SWEET TOOTH

The natural way for satisfying our sweet tooth is to eat sweet fruits. Dried fruits, such as dates, figs, and raisins are especially desirable. Dried fruits and the juice of sweet fruits can also be substituted successfully in many delicious dessert recipes. In moderation, there are many simple sugars derived from plants and found in many whole foods markets worldwide that can healthfully satisfy our craving for sweets. Some of the most common are highlighted as follows:

Barley Malt Syrup. Sprouted, roasted barley that has been slow-cooked with water to make a thick syrup. It is a pleasant sweetener that can be used in most baked goods, but is especially recommended for bread-baking.

Brown Rice Syrup. Brown rice that has been cooked for such a long time that it liquifies. It has a light, sweet taste and is a great addition to delicate desserts, especially for people suffering from food allergies.

Date and Fig Syrups. These have been used as sweeteners for thousands of years. Today they are made commercially through a mechanical process that pulverizes the raw dates or figs and mixes them with water. Date sugar can be found in many food markets. Date sugar comes from dried dates which have been pulverized into crystals to form date sugar.

Honey (raw). A thick sweet liquid produced by bees and stored in honeycombs. Raw honey that is not commercially processed is a powerhouse of nutrients. One tablespoon of raw honey contains about 50 mg. of calcium, 200 mg. of potassium, 20 mg. of magnesium, 25 mg. of iron, 2.4 mg. of B-1, 1.2 mg of B-2, and 3 mg. of niacin. Compare these nutrient levels to most commercial sweeteners, such as table sugar, which contain just empty calories.

Maple Sugar and Maple Syrup. The result of a boiling process that reduces large quantities of maple sap into a concentrated syrupy "sugar" called pure maple syrup. If maple syrup is boiled down until it becomes a soft, granular sugar, it is called maple sugar. Maple syrup is great in hot drinks and on cereal and pancakes. It is also versatile and may be used successfully in baked goods like muffins, cookies, and cakes, especially if blended with the more nutrient dense unsulphured molasses. Be careful when buying maple syrup. It should say pure Maple Syrup on the food label. Otherwise, it could be mixed with undesirable refined sugars such as corn syrup. Maple syrup is also a great choice from those suffering from grain allergies.

Molasses (unsulphured). The liquid removed from sugar cane before processing. It contains a decent amount of potassium, calcium, magnesium, and iron. Because it has a strong taste, it is best mixed with other sweeteners, such as pure maple syrup.

Prune puree. This can be made from pulverized prunes that have been mixed with water. It is great for cooking and baking because it can be used to replace most of the fat in baked goods while still maintaining moisture. It tastes great and is also one of nature's best laxatives! Many food markets are now stocking prune puree (it is usually labeled as a fat and egg substitute under the brand name Wonderslim™).

Stevia. Derived from the powdered leaf of an intensely sweet South American herb with the same name. Its sweetness comes from glucoside, which our bodies cannot completely metabolize, thus making it essentially non-caloric. Stevia is used as a sweetener in many countries, such as Japan, and has no history of side effects. In fact, some scientific research has indicated that it can help balance blood glucose levels. Stevia was approved as a non-caloric sweetener by the FDA in 1996; but unfortunately, due to political pressure from the manufacturers of other non-caloric sweeteners, it cannot as yet be added to products such as diet foods and soft drinks. It can be found in natural foods markets as a dietary supplement.

Sucanat. A dehydrated, organically grown cane juice that still retains its trace nutrients such as Vitamin A and potassium. It may be used in place of brown sugar because it has a similar mouth feel and taste. Sucanat is currently being studied for safety for diabetics.

Juice. Derived from any sweet fruit or vegetable, may be substituted for refined sugar in most recipes. Frozen concentrated juices work best because they are firmer and sweeter. Use frozen juice concentrates in gelatins, milk-free shakes, frozen yogurt, and pie recipes.

FIBER

No discussion of carbohydrates would be complete without mentioning the importance of fiber. Paleolithic man ate a high amount of insoluble and soluble fiber coming primarily from nuts and seeds, berries, root vegetables, and wild grasses.

A high fiber diet not only optimizes the elimination process and transit time, but also supports the growth of lactobacilli and other friendly flora in the large intestine while inhibiting disease-causing bacteria and parasites from attaching themselves to the intestinal lining. High fiber diets have been shown to reduce cholesterol levels, protect against colon cancer, regulate fluctuating blood sugar levels, and optimize digestion.

It is preferable to get fiber from dietary sources. Too many people rely on insoluble, allergenic or inflammatory substances like whole wheat and psyllium husks for their sole source(s) of fiber. As with all foods, variety and moderation are necessary. I recommend 15–30 grams of fiber daily to most of my clients from the following optimum sources:

Type of Fiber	Amount	Fiber (grams)
Bread and Crackers		
Barley (cooked)	½ cup	2.2
Corn Bran	½ cup	4.4
Corn Flakes	¾ cup	2.6
Oatmeal	¾ pkg.	2.5
Oat Bran	¾ cup	4.5
Pumpernickel bread	¾ slice	1.4
Quinoa (cooked)	½ cup	6.0
Rice, brown (cooked)	½ cup	2.4
Rice, wild (cooked)	½ cup	3.2
Rice, white (cooked)	½ cup	.75
Rye bread	1 slice	.8
Rye crackers	3 large	5
Sprouted Whole Grain bread	1 slice	5.0
Fruit		
Apple	½ large	2.0
Apricot	2	1.4
Banana	½ medium	1.5
Blackberries	¾ cup	6.7

Type of Fiber	Amount	Fiber (grams)
Fruit *(continued)*		
Blueberries	¾ cup	8.0
Cantaloupe	1 cup	1.6
Cherries	10 large	1.1
Dates, dried	2	1.6
Grapefruit	½	0.8
Honeydew melon	1 cup	1.5
Orange	1 small	1.6
Peach	1 medium	2.3
Pineapple	½	0.8
Plum	3 small	1.8
Prunes, dried	2	2.4
Raisins	1.5 Tbs.	1.0
Raspberries	¾ cup	8.0
Strawberries	1 cup	3.0
Tangerine	1 large	2.0
Watermelon	1 cup	1.4
Rice		
Rice, brown (cooked)	½ cup	2.4
Rice, white (cooked)	½ cup	.75
Vegetables		
Broccoli	½ cup	3.5
Brussels sprouts	½ cup	2.3
Cabbage	½ cup	2.1
Cauliflower	½ cup	1.6
Celery	½ cup	1.1
Lettuce	1 cup	0.8
Spinach, raw	1 cup	0.2
Turnip greens	½ cup	3.5
Beets	½ cup	2.1
Carrots	½ cup	2.4
Potatoes, sweet, baked	½ medium	2.1
Potatoes, white, baked (no skin)	½ medium	1.9
Potatoes, white, baked (with skin)	½ medium	5
Radishes	½ cup	1.3
Peas, green	¾ cup	4.0

Type of Fiber	Amount	Fiber (grams)
Vegetables *(continued)*		
Beans, string	¾ cup	3.0
Cucumber	¾ cup	1.75
Eggplant	¾ cup	4.0
Legumes (red, white, black beans; lentils, soybeans, chick peas)	¾ cup	7–10
Onions	½ cup	1.2
Tomatoes	1 small	1.5
Winter squash, acorn	½ medium	5
Zucchini squash	¾ cup	3.0

There are basically seven types of fiber:

Cellulose. An indigestible carbohydrate, it is found in fruits and vegetables, the outer shells of whole grains, and the bark of trees (methycellulose, a non-allergenic source of added fiber)

Gums. Resin-like, sticky substances, these are found in many plants (guar gum, agar)

Lignans. Found in large amounts in Brazil nuts, white potatoes, peas and other legumes

Pectin. The fiber is found in large amounts in apples, citrus fruits, carrots, and okra

Hemicellulose. Found in large amounts in apples, bananas, legumes, green leafy vegetables, cabbage, and whole grains is another form of indigestible fiber

Mucliages. Sticky substances found in plants such as flaxseed, mucilages may have a cholesterol lowering benefit and stabilize erratic blood sugar levels

Brans. Found in the outer casings of whole grains, these are bulking agents that may benefit in lowering total and LDL cholesterol levels

Personal Case Study #5

Carbo-loading, especially with grains, has been one of the biggest nutritional changes in the U.S. in the last five years. One just needs to look at the USDA Food Pyramid on a cereal package or the number of bread and bagel stores popping up nationwide to realize that the American public is obsessed with grains.

Bill P., a 46 year old pre-diabetic of Italian heritage, was shocked when I told him that he was eating at least three times his ideal carbo intake, especially from bread and pasta. He asked me how carbos could be so bad when even the U.S. Department of Agriculture recommends 6–11 servings of grains daily with 3–5 vegetables and 2–4 fruits (all carbos). I explained that the Food Pyramid hasn't been effective because in the last few years, Americans have become fatter and sicker than at any other time in history. If he wanted to prevent diabetes and obesity he had to cut his bread, pasta and total carbo intake dramatically.

As with most of my clients, cutting out breads was the most difficult task; but after six weeks, he did not even miss them anymore when delicious smells wafted from the bread basket at his favorite Italian restaurant. His triglycerides and blood sugar were back to normal within three months. It also did not hurt that 22 fat pounds came right off of his mid-section. He raved about the fact that he had the same pants size now as he did when he married 20 years ago! I asked him if he still missed bread. His response was, "As long as I have it only occasionally," (his favorite cheating strategy was to dip delicious bread crust into olive oil sprinkled with Parmesan Cheese), "I can control my weight and blood sugar. That and my renewed energy does not make avoiding bread a sacrifice."

TABLE I
FOOD VALUES OF SWEETENERS

N = Natural Sugar   R = Refined Sugar

Measures		White Granulated Sugar (R)	Powdered Sugar (R)	Sugar in the Raw (unbleached) (R)	Sucanat (unrefined evaporated cane juice) (N)	Light Brown Sugar (caramel colored) (R)	Date Sugar (pulverized dates) (N)	Blackstrap Molasses (N)	Raw Honey (strained) (N)	Commercial Honey (R)	Corn Syrup (R)	Pure Maple Syrup (N)	Apple Juice (frozen concentrate) (N)
Measure	1 T.	1 T.	1 T.	1 T.	1 T.	1 T.	1 T.	1 T.	1 T.	1 T.	1 T.	1 T.	
Weight	(gm)	12	11	14	13	13	11.1	20	21	21	20	20	29.9
Calories		46	42	33	30	48	30.6	43	52	64	57	50	13.9
Carbohydrate	(gm)	11.9	10.9	12.7	6.99	12.6	8.1	11	11	17.8	14.8	12.8	3.5
Protein	(gm)	0	0	0	0	0	Tr.	0	0	0	0	0	Tr.
Sodium	(mg)	0	0	0	0	0	0	20	18	1	30	3	2.1
Calcium	(mg)	0	0	7	8	0	6.6	137	49	4	9	33	1.8
Phosphorus	(mg)	0	0	6	2.3	0	7	17	35	1	3	3	1
Potassium	(mg)	0	0	0	47	0	72.1	585	205	11	0	26	19
Magnesium	(mg)	0	0	0	6	0	2.9	51.6	19	0.6	0	0	.8
Iron	(mg)	0	0	0.6	0.3	0	Tr.	3.2	25	0.1	0.8	0.6	Tr.
Thiamine-B1	(mg)	0	0	Tr.	Tr.	0	Tr.	Tr.	2.4	Tr.	0	0	0
Riboflv.-B2	(mg)	0	0	0	Tr.	0	Tr.	Tr.	1.2	Tr.	Tr.	0	0
Niacin	(mg)	0	0	0	Tr.	0	0.2	0.4	3	0.1	0	0	Tr.
Vitamin A	(IU)	0	0	Tr.	77	0	5.6	0	0	0	0	0	0
Vitamin C	(mg)	0	0	0.3	2.3	0	0	0	3	Tr.	0.1	0	Tr.
Folic Acid	(mcg)	0	0	0	—	0	1	2	15	1	0	0	Tr.

Sources:

Food Values of Portions Commonly Used. Pennington & Church. 14th Ed., 1985

Nutrition Almanac. Nutrition Search, Inc. 2nd Ed., 1984.

Nutritive Value of Foods. U.S. Dept. of Agriculture. April, 1981.

TABLE II

NATURAL SWEETENERS TO REPLACE ONE CUP OF SUGAR

Sweetener	Amount to Replace the Sweetness in 1 cup of Sugar	Liquid Reduction Needed	Suggested Use
Barley malt	1 to 1½ cups	¼ cup	– baking
Brown rice syrup	1 to 1½ cups	¼ cup	– baking
Date sugar	⅔ cup	—	– cooking/baking
Honey or fig syrup	¾ cup	⅛ cup	– all purpose; fruit pies and other fruit desserts; "Jello"
Juice concentrate	1 to 1½ cups	½ cup	
Maple syrup	¾ cup	¼ cup	– baking
Maple sugar	½ to ⅔ cup	—	– candy
Molasses	½ cup	¼ cup	– baking (with other sweeteners
Prune puree	½ cup	¼ cup	– baking
Sucanat	1 cup	—	– all purpose; baking

TABLE III

FRESH JUICES..."NECTAR OF THE GODS"

Please Note: Each recipe yields 8-12 ounces of juice.

Carrot Apple Juice

4 carrots, medium size
2 Granny Smith apples, cored & peeled
and blend
Blend all ingredients in a juicer or Cuisinart.

Berry Good Drink

2 apples, cored and peeled
1 pint strawberries
1 pint raspberries
Blend all ingredients in a juicer or Cuisinart.

Dr. Nieper's Cleansing Cocktail

4 carrots
1 apple, cored and peeled
2 pieces of celery, leaves removed
several garlic cloves
1/2 beet with tops
Blend all ingredients in a juicer or cuisinart.

Kiwi Apple

2 Granny Smith apples, cored and peeled
3 kiwi, peeled

Blend the apples and kiwi in a juicer or Cuisinart.

Ginger Ale (great for digestion)

1/4 inch piece of ginger
1 lemon wedge
1 apple, cored and peeled
4 oz. sparkling mineral water

Put the first three ingredients in a juicer or cuisinart. Add the water and blend again until smooth.

Anti-Cholesterol Cocktail

1/4 inch of ginger, peeled
1 clove garlic
Handful of parsley
1 apple, cored and peeled

Put all ingredients in a cuisinart or juicer in the order listed. Blend until smooth.

Carrot Jicama Apple

4 carrots
1 medium jicama, peeled
1 apple, cored and peeled

Blend all ingredients in a cuisinart or juicer.

Passion Drink

2 pieces passion fruit
2 lemons
2 kiwi

Blend all ingredients in a cuisinart or juicer.

Femme Fatale—Aphrodisiac

1 small head of fennel
2 apples, cored and peeled
2 ribs of celery, leaves removed

Blend all ingredients in a cuisinart or juicer.

Stevia Extract may be added to any recipe for added sweetness.

Some recipes adapted from *A Complete Book of Juicing* by Michael T. Murray

ᴄ 6 ᴐ

The Skinny on Fats

The world is obsessed with the consumption of dietary fat. Many Americans who want to lose weight have a fear of consuming any dietary fat. They count fat grams from every food they eat and avoid fat like the plague. In many third-world countries, people are desperate to find enough fat just to stay alive. Although these two diverse populations appear to be at opposite ends of the spectrum, both groups are in the fat starvation mode, which is causing them physical harm.

The human body craves and needs dietary fat. Dietary fat is often referred to as "essential fatty acids." Without fat we cannot absorb the fat soluble vitamins A, E, D, and K from the foods we eat. Fat is also essential for supplying us with a constant source of energy, and is especially helpful in providing us with energy reserves in times of illness or famine. Fat helps keep us warm in cold weather, slows down digestion of foods in the gastrointestinal tract to give us a feeling of fullness, and increases flavor in the foods we eat.

Excess consumption of all dietary fats can cause weight gain because every gram of fat contains nine calories. There are only four calories for every gram of protein or carbohydrate. When you eat foods that are high in fat, you will be ingesting more than double the calories you would be consuming from protein or carbohydrate foods. High fat foods are always high calorie foods. The average American consumes as many as 40–50% of daily calories from fat. It is important to choose fats wisely and in moderation because a diet high in fat (usually more than 20–30% of daily calories) increases your risk for obesity, digestive disorders, heart disease, diabetes, gallbladder problems, and certain types of cancer.

Most dietary fats in the U.S. come from animals. The fat content of meat, if too high, causes health risks. We know from archeological research that all wild and grazing animals in ancient times were much leaner than are the caged, chemically fed, unexercised animals found in most commercial markets in the U.S. today. Animal by-products (milk and eggs) would also have contained less fat and cholesterol in ancient times than they do today.

The American Heart Association's recommendation for consuming 30% or less of our daily calories from dietary fat does not show the complete picture. Saturated fats, which come primarily from red meat, palm and coconut oils cause the most serious health risks. The "fat" problem associated with milk products, eggs, and poultry today (especially in the United States), is directly caused by the fat-producing feed, drugs, (especially antibiotics and hormones), and lack of exercise given to animals. Not only were ancient animal food sources lower in saturated fat and cholesterol than they are today, but they were also free of the harmful drug and pesticide residues that may be contributing to the high rates of breast and other hormonally related cancers. Fortunately, free range, organic, and Kosher sources of animal products contain no harmful additives. In many cases, they also contain less total fat, but especially less saturated fat.

There is a common misconception that dietary cholesterol is always harmful and that it causes high blood cholesterol levels. Research, such as the ongoing Framingham Heart Studies, has proven that dietary cholesterol levels do not cause high cholesterol levels. The culprit is dietary **saturated fat**. While certain types of fats are beneficial for ideal blood cholesterol levels, others are harmful.

Cholesterol has an important purpose in maintaining human health. When we are faced with illness or extreme stress, our bodies produce cholesterol to give us a feeling of well-being. Cholesterol levels that are too low (usually a total below 130) create very low energy and have now been implicated in cancer, depression, and suicide. We're not sure if the lower cholesterol is a cause or result of these serious health risks. Ideal cholesterol levels, according to Framingham, are shown in Table II.

Fish are rarely farmed commercially so are more closely related to the fat content in fish eaten throughout history. The omega 3 fatty acids found in fish have been scientifically proven to be the heart healthiest, most cancer-preventing fats known if their swimming waters have not been polluted by mercury, lead, PCB's or other toxic, man-made pollutants.

Table I lists and compares the main categories of dietary fats which include saturated fats, hydrogenated fats, polyunsaturated fats, monounsaturated fats, and the omega 3 fatty acids. Following are definitions of these fats:

Saturated fats.   These can be easily identified because they will remain solid at room temperature. These fats provide the most health risks to humans. Ideally, less than 10% of our daily food intake should come from saturated fats. Chief sources of fats are meat, dairy products, lard, and tropical oils (coconut, palm, and cocoa butter). Saturated fats may increase the risk of serious health problems such as heart disease and stroke by increasing blood cholesterol levels (especially, the bad "LDL" cholesterol) and building up plaque in the arteries.

Hydrogenated fats.   For at least the last decade, these were touted as healthy. They have now been found to cause more severe health problems than do most saturated fats. The process of hydrogenation totally changes the molecular structure of a fat, which prevents the human body from metabolizing it in a safe way.

This process became popular mainly to prevent fats from turning rancid. Margarine, which is almost always hydrogenated, will remain solid at room temperature because it has become saturated. The saturated **trans** fatty acids that are formed during the process of hydrogenation have a much higher risk of causing coronary artery disease. For example, a Harvard study published in Lancet (March, 1993) found that women who consumed foods high in **trans** fatty acids, especially from margarine, had a 50% higher risk for coronary artery disease than did women who consumed these fats rarely! Another study, reported in the *American Journal of Cardiology* (April, 1993), concluded that people with diagnosed heart disease had very high levels of trans fatty acids in their blood. Health "experts" who still recommend margarine over butter, in light of this negative research, are doing a disservice to the public. At least butter is a "real" food, with thousands of years of recorded consumption. The key to consumption of butter or any saturated fat is "moderation."

Hydrogenated fats should be avoided completely. Besides margarine, other common sources of these "manmade" fats include packaged snack chips, crackers, cupcakes, and candy bars.

Polyunsaturated fats. These remain liquid at room temperature. If refrigerated, they should only make up 10% or less of the human diet. Polyunsaturates are found primarily in sunflower, safflower, corn, and soybean oils. These fats were highly recommended in the United States until recent research uncovered problems such as lowering the good "HDL" cholesterol while lowering total cholesterol. Also, at least one of these fats, namely corn oil, has been linked to cancer if consumed in large amounts.

Monounsaturated fats. Liquid at room temperature, they may or may not become solid if refrigerated. They come primarily from olives, nuts, seeds, and avocados. These are the healthiest fats (canola, olive, peanut, nut, and avocado oils). Mediterraneans, who generally consume more than 30% of their daily calories from monounsaturated fats, are some of the heart-healthiest people in the world. Research has proven that even in generous amounts, monounsaturated fats have been shown to protect the heart by raising the good "HDL" cholesterol while lowering the bad "LDL" cholesterol.

Also, monounsaturated fats help cleanse the digestive tract and aid in elimination.

I would like to say a few words about the much maligned **avocado**. It is banned like the plague for most weight loss diets. This is a real shame because avocados are very high in monounsaturated fat (see Table I) and also contain healthy amounts of potassium, magnesium, B-6, Vitamin C, and zinc. Recent research has even shown avocados to stabilize blood sugar levels among both hypoglycemic and diabetic individuals.

Ideally, monounsaturated fats should be consumed as the primary fat source on a daily basis. Delicious ways of adding this type of fat are a handful of raw nuts and seeds for breakfast, avocado on a salad for lunch, and olive oil in cooking or as a salad dressing for dinner.

Omega 3 fatty acids. Found in generous amounts in fish and to a lesser extent in flax and rapeseed (canola oil), they have been shown in scientific studies to help prevent heart disease by preventing platelets from forming clots so that arteries will not be blocked. Cold water, fatty fish (i.e. salmon, halibut, mackerel) are a rich source of Omega 3 fatty acids and should ideally be consumed at least three times a week. A recent Yale study indicated that eating only eight ounces of fish per week can cut the risk of having a heart attack by half! For those individuals who do not eat fish, an Omega 3 dietary supplement in capsule form may be warranted (although some people report headaches from fish oil supplements). Regular consumption of flax seeds or oil (which is now being studied as a colon cancer preventative) and/or canola oil will also provide small amounts of these essential Omega 3 fats.

Just the Facts about Fat

Modern man could have saved decades of suffering through the "fat issue" if experts had simply paid attention to what ancient man ate. If we consume mostly monounsaturated fats and saturated fats in moderation as have our ancestors for thousands of years, we should not have to be afraid of fats. The American obesity problem has skyrocketed in the past ten years. We are the fattest nation in the world and are heavier right now than at any other time in history. Our obesity problem is not only due to eating too much added fat, but to eating too many total calories, too many fake foods, choosing the worst fats, and substituting too many grains and simple carbo-hydrates for dietary fat.

Personal Case Study #6

Michael M. was an obese 29 year old construction work-er. A blood test showed a total cholesterol of 335, with an LDL cholesterol of 263 and an HDL of 29. He was a fast food aficionado—doughnuts and coffee for breakfast, burger, fries and large cola for lunch, and fried chicken, mashed potatoes, coleslaw, and sugar-laden iced tea with a few beers for dinner. His doctor told him he was a "heart attack waiting to happen." Michael tried several heart medications at the insistence of his cardiologist, but each one caused symptoms of lack of libido, increased liver enzymes, spaciness or all three. Against his doctor's wishes, he finally refused further medication and came to see me.

Michael had been put on a diet where everything was fat free. This regimen showed a gradual weight loss, but for the last few months he was cranky and irritable. He also had a grayish pallor and said he was always starving. I recommended 2–3 daily servings of healthy fats (espe-cially olive oil, sunflower seeds, salmon, almonds and avocado), fewer carbohydrates and more lean animal protein (especially fish, turkey and chicken in that order). Within two weeks his ravenous appetite diminished and his energy level increased. The addition of heart healthy nutrients (Magnesium, B-6, B-12, Folic Acid, Vitamin E and CoQ10) gave him the incentive to make major dietary improvements and stick with them long term.

His cardiologist was amazed when three months

after our first appointment Michael's total cholesterol was 192, his LDL was 117 and his HDL was 53. He had lost 26 pounds and had gained muscle mass. Michael was so relieved and shocked by such a change without medication that he asked his cardiologist why he had not prescribed supplemental nutrients and a dietary change instead of medications. The cardiologist shrugged his shoulders and said "we were not taught nutrition in medical school, and **most people** will not change their eating habits anyway." Fortunately, Michael was not "most people."

TABLE I

COMPARISON OF DIETARY FATS

Plant oils contain 120 calories and 13–15 grams of fat per tablespoon. Stick butter is 100 calories and about 11.5 grams of fat per tablespoon, whipped butter is 60 calories and 7 grams of fat per tablespoon, and lard is 115 calories and 13 grams of fat per tablespoon. Choose the fats, most often, that contain the highest amount of monounsaturated fat and the lowest amount of saturated fat.

Type of Fat	Monounsaturated (in grams)	Polyunsaturated (in grams)	Saturated (in grams)
Almond	10	2	1
Avocado	10	2	2
Butter, stick	3	1	7
Canola (rapeseed)	8	4	1
Coconut	1	—	12
Corn	3	8	2
Cottonseed	2	7	4
Lard (animal tallow)	4	2	7
Margarine, stick	5	4	(hydrogenated) 2
Olive	10	1	2
Palm	5	1	7
Palm kernel	2	—	11
Peanut	6	5	2
Safflower	2	10	1
Sesame	5	6	2
Soybean	3	8	2
Sunflower	3	9	1
Walnut	3	9	1

Foods High in Omega 3 fatty acids listed in order from most to least:
Fish (especially high-fat varieties such as salmon)
Flax oil
Leafy greens (especially purslane)
Canola oil
Soybean oil
Walnut oil
Pumpkin seeds

Sources:
Center for Genetics, Nutrition and Health, Washington D.C., 1991
University of California at Berkeley Wellness Letter, September 1993
U.S. Department of Agriculture, 1991

TABLE II

NATIONAL CHOLESTEROL EDUCATION PROGRAM FRAMINGHAM HEART INSTITUTE CUTOFFS

Constituent	Desirable	Borderline	Unfavorable
Cholesterol	*LT 200 mg/dl	200-239 mg/dl	GT/EQ 240 mg/dl
LDL	LT 130 mg/dl	130-159 mg/dl	GT/EQ 160 mg/dl
HDL	*GT 50 mg/dl	LT 45 mg/dl	LT 35 mg/dl
LDL/HDL	LT 3.22	GT 3.22	GT 5.03
CHOL/HDL	LT 4.44	GT 4.44	GT 7.05

*Please note:
LT means less than.
GT means greater than.

ᴝ 7 ᴝ

Nutritional Supplements

According to a report in the May 1997 issue of *The Western Journal of Medicine*, significant reductions could be made in the number of recorded birth defects, premature births and instances of coronary heart disease with daily vitamin and mineral intake. The report also states that dramatic dollar savings (as much as $20 billion each year) could be made with regular use of specific nutrient supplements. Taking dietary supplements indiscriminately is not recommended. Vitamin and mineral benefits are highlighted in this section. The top ten supplements for optimum health are explained in detail.

VITAMINS AND MINERALS
(MICRONUTRIENTS NECESSARY TO SUSTAIN LIFE)

Although eating a well-balanced diet of wholesome, nutrient-dense foods is important, an optimal and consistent intake of vitamins and minerals in supplement form will ensure that our body will function at its best. A single deficiency of a vitamin or mineral can adversely impact our body. The vitamin and mineral micronutrients in foods and most supplement formulas are as follows:

VITAMINS

Vitamin A. A fat-soluble vitamin that strengthens the immune system; promotes healthy eyes, skin and healthy mucus membranes. Ideal Food Sources: fish liver oils (cod liver oil); green, yellow, orange, and red fruits and vegetables (high in carotenoids).

Vitamin C. A powerful antioxidant; protects cell from damage caused by free radicals; supports the immune system; essential for collagen and connective tissue formation; enhances healing. Ideal Food Sources: citrus fruits, kiwi, berries; small amounts in most fruits and vegetables.

Vitamin D. A fat-soluble vitamin that regulates calcium balance and absorption; aids in healthy bone and teeth formation; strengthens the immune system. Ideal Food Sources: fish liver oils (cod liver oil), fatty saltwater fish such as halibut, salmon, and sardines; fortified dairy, soymilk, and rice milk; egg yolks. *Please note: the best source of absorbable Vitamin D comes from sunlight exposure to the skin.*

Vitamin E.   A powerful antioxidant. A fat-soluble vitamin that enhances nervous system function; helps prevent blood clots; reduces pain from varicose veins and fibrocystic breasts. Ideal Food Sources: cold-pressed vegetable oils; nuts/seeds (cold-pressed nut/seed oils); whole grains.

Vitamin K.   A fat-soluble vitamin essential for normal blood clotting, bone formation and bone repair. Ideal Food Sources: dark green leafy vegetables; egg yolks; liver. *Please note: the best source of Vitamin K is synthesized internally in the body's intestines by "friendly" bacteria.*

B COMPLEX

Vitamin B-1. (Thiamine) Allows protein, carbohydrate, and fat to produce energy; helps with detoxification of harmful substances; enhances nervous system function. Ideal Food Sources: brown rice, egg yolks, legumes, fish, pork, and poultry.

Vitamin B-2. (Riboflavin) Important for cellular energy; supports hormone production; helps with neurotransmission; helps produce healthy red blood cells, eyes and skin. Ideal Food Sources: egg yolks, fish, red meat, poultry, spinach, yogurt, and cheese.

Vitamin B-3. (Niacin) Allows protein, carbohydrate, and fat to be absorbed and utilized for energy; synthesizes fats and regulates certain hormones; aids in the formation of red blood cells. Ideal Food Sources: beef liver, eggs, fish, pork, broccoli, dates, tomatoes, and potatoes.

Vitamin B-6. (Pyridoxine) Important for protein synthesis; helps to manufacture hormones, red blood cells and enzymes; important for a healthy immune system (especially in prevention of allergic reactions); helps to regulate hormones and brain function; removes excess fluid; reduces homocysteine levels (a risk factor for heart disease). Ideal Food Sources: chicken, eggs, red meat, peas, spinach, sunflower seeds, most nuts (especially walnuts).

Vitamin B-12. (Cyanocobalamin) Supports the health of the nervous system and the development and utilization of red blood cells; important for digestion and absorption of food; energizes the cells; reduces homocysteine levels (a risk factor for heart disease). Ideal Food Sources: bioavailable sources are found only in animal foods, especially liver, fish, shellfish, yogurt, and cheese.

Pantothenic Acid. Important for the breakdown of fats, carbohydrates, and protein to produce energy; assists in the production of fats, cholesterol, bile, Vitamin D, neurotransmitters and adrenal gland hormones.

Biotin. Assists energy metabolism; promotes healthy skin, hair, and mucus membranes. Ideal Food Sources: egg yolks, red meat, poultry, saltwater fish, soybeans, and whole grains.

Folic Acid. Regulates cell division and transfer of inherited traits from the mother and father to the fetus; prevents neural tube defects; supports healthy gums, red blood cells, skin, the gastrointestinal tract, and the immune system; reduces homocysteine levels (a risk for heart disease). Ideal Food Sources: barley, beef, pork, brown rice, salmon, tuna, oranges, peas, chicken, and fortified grains.

Choline. Aids lipid balance by assisting in the production and transportation of fats from the liver; supports normal nerve and brain function. Ideal Food Sources: egg yolks, soy lecithin, legumes.

Inositol. Assists fat metabolism as a partner to choline; aids in nerve transmission and the regulation of certain enzymes. Ideal Food Sources: soy lecithin, legumes, raisins, small amounts in many fruits and vegetables.

MINERALS

Calcium. Essential for the development and maintenance of healthy bones and teeth; important for electrolyte balance, optimizes blood pressure and health of cell membranes. Ideal Food Sources: yogurt, cheese, salmon, sardines, shellfish, nuts/seeds, dark green leafy vegetables (especially dandelion greens, beet greens, kale, spinach); fortified orange juice, soy products, and rice milk.

Magnesium. May be the most important nutrient because it is a catalyst for most body functions including muscle and heart metabolism, synthesis of genetic material within each cell, nerve transmission and relaxation, and the conversion of carbohydrates, proteins, and fats to energy; approximately 72% of all adult Americans are deficient in magnesium intake and/or absorption. Ideal Food Sources: avocados, kiwi, nuts/seeds, soy products, bananas, oranges, salmon, halibut, mackerel, unsulphured and blackstrap molasses.

Boron. Assists in the absorption of calcium and building of strong bones. Ideal Food Sources: leafy vegetables, nuts, pears, grapes, apples, carrots.

Iron. Carries oxygen into the blood and regulates oxygen in all cellular tissue; supports the immune system; allows the body to maintain energy and optimum brain function. (Should not be taken in supplement form of more than 10 mg. daily by most men and post-menopausal women.) Ideal Food Sources: liver, red meat, unsulphured and blackstrap molasses, raisins, dried apricots, fortified cereals.

Copper. Plays a role in the absorption and release of iron; aids in the conversion of nutrients to energy; helps to maintain the cardiovascular and skeletal systems; helps to balance zinc. Ideal Food Sources: almonds, avocados, barley, broccoli, garlic, chocolate (cocoa powder)

Zinc. Important for protein synthesis; is a component of many enzyme functions; regulates blood sugar and brain function; necessary for growth, sexual function, healing, and reproduction; maintains health of skin, immune system and digestive tract; regulates appetite and hunger; important for the senses of taste and smell. Ideal Food Sources: fish, shellfish, seaweed, kelp, red meats, nuts/seeds (especially sunflower seeds), eggs, soy products.

Manganese. Important for the formation of connective tissue and bone; necessary for energy production, reproduction, and glucose metabolism. Ideal Food Sources: avocados, nuts/seeds, seaweed, whole grains.

Chromium. Necessary for blood sugar balance; assists in building muscle and burning body fat. Ideal Food Sources: brown rice, red meat, whole grains, cheese.

Selenium. A powerful antioxidant and cancer preventative. Ideal Food Sources: brazil nuts, broccoli, brown rice, garlic, onions, kelp, salmon, shellfish, tuna, whole grains.

Molybdenum. Important for the utilization of iron; necessary for normal growth and development; a catalyst for several enzyme functions. Ideal Food Sources: legumes, cereal grains, dark green leafy vegetables.

Potassium. Important for muscle expansion and contraction; assists in nerve conduction; regulates heartbeat and electrolytes in conjunction with magnesium.

Ideal Food Sources: bananas, avocados, kiwi; unsulphured and blackstrap molasses; poultry; salmon, halibut, mackerel; white potatoes; nuts/seeds.

Iodine. Necessary for physical and mental development; needed for a healthy thyroid gland and goiter prevention; Ideal Food Sources: iodized salt, saltwater fish, shellfish, kelp, sea salt, garlic, mineral water.

TOP TEN SUPPLEMENTS:

1. MAGNESIUM
(MAGNESIUM GLYCINATE—PATENT #4,830,716)

According to recent Hanes and Gallop surveys, at least 72% of all adult Americans fall short of the United States recommended dietary allowance for magnesium. Serum (blood) magnesium levels are not an accurate test for total body stores of this mineral because magnesium is primarily a cellular mineral. Also, stress depletes this mineral rapidly. Thus, supplementing magnesium is recommended for all adult Americans.

Magnesium is a catalyst for at least 30 organ functions. Some of its benefits include:
1. protein synthesis,
2. regulation of the parathyroid hormone release which regulates bone calcification,
3. cellular respiration,
4. nerve transmission,
5. prostaglandin synthesis,
6. cardiac muscle health,
7. female hormone balance.

According to Melvin Werbach, M.D., Professor at UCLA School of Medicine, some of the most alarming magnesium deficiency symptoms which are rarely diagnosed by the medical profession relate to the following disorders: hypotension, hypertension, kidney stones, muscular weakness, neuromuscular irritability, hemolytic anemia, bronchial asthma, organic brain syndrome, eclampsia of pregnancy, migraine headaches, tachycardia, cardiac arrhythmia, myocardial infarction, edema, hyper-kinetic behavior, insomnia, severe muscle pain, seizures, vertigo, chronic fatigue syndrome, diabetes, coarse muscle tremors, osteoporosis, psychiatric disorders, shortness of breath, and poor pulmonary function.

Most Americans cannot get enough magnesium from diet alone. Unfortunately, most supplemental magnesium comes in oxide, aspartate, sulfate, or hydrochloride forms which can cause diarrhea and abdominal cramps among sensitive individuals. Magnesium Glycinate, on the other hand, is a patented (U.S. Patent #4,830,716) revolutionary process of chelating magnesium to glycine so that the magnesium is absorbed like an amino acid. It is so well absorbed that it is not dependent on stomach acid or diet. It is released easily into target organs for higher absorption and nutrient density.

2. CALCIUM (MICROCRYSTALLINE HYDROXAPATITE)

Calcium is one of the most essential nutrients for maintaining bone health, but one of the most misunderstood by health professionals. Contrary to a common misconception, bone is a living substance! In fact, bone is one of the most active tissues in the body. It is constantly being dissolved and rebuilt in a process called remodeling and, like any other living tissue, needs nourishment to stay strong and healthy. Besides building strong bones, calcium is also essential for maintenance of a regular heartbeat, transmission of nerve impulses, proper muscular contraction, activation of several enzymes (including lipase), and proper cell membrane permeability.

However, excess calcium (especially from calcium carbonate or dairy products), a milk allergy or lactose intolerance, can cause improper absorption of calcium causing kidney stones, bone and heel spurs, fibrocystic breasts, and joint pain. Most calcium supplements have very poor absorption rates because the sources are not complete bone foods (i.e. citrate, aspartate, chelate, ascorbate, lactate, and carbonate). Calcium carbonate, in particular, will almost always be malabsorbed by elderly people due to its antacid effect. Stomach acid is essential for absorption of calcium, and because older people tend to have less stomach acid, calcium carbonate interferes with protein digestion and can cause gas, bloating, and constipation. Bone meal is a complete bone food, but, according to recent testing, has been found to contain high levels of toxic metals (i.e. arsenic, lead, cadmium). There has been a national alert for the public to avoid bone meal as a dietary supplement. Thus, we are left with MCHC (Microcrystalline Hydroxapatite Concentrate), the most complete bone food that's safe from toxic substances, well absorbed, and has been shown repeatedly to reduce bone loss and restore lost bone.

Microcrystalline hydroxyapatite concentrate (MCHC) is whole bone extract and is now available as a nutritional supplement. It provides much greater nourishment than just calcium. MCHC contains protein and other ingredients that comprise the organic portion of bone, as well as calcium and other minerals in the normal physiological proportions found in raw bone.

Numerous case studies of individuals switching from heavy dairy product intake and/or incomplete bone food supplements to MCHC have shown that if taken in a dosage of 1,000–1,500 mg. daily this supplementation has resulted in rapid restoration of broken bones and improvement in significant bone density (3–7% per year) even among osteoporotic females. The best supplemented calcium for most people over the age of 45 is MCHC.

3. Antioxidants: Carnitine, CoQ10, and ACES

Carnitine, also referred to as Acetyl L-Carnitine, is responsible for transporting fats into the mitochondria where they can then be converted to energy. L-Carnitine is found in the brain, but its levels are dramatically reduced as we age. Recent studies have identified L-Carnitine as one of the most significant anti-aging compounds for the brain and nervous system. It can prevent neuron death due to its release and synthesis of choline.

In addition to Carnitine's energizing and neuron protecting effects, it also has been shown to dramatically reduce cardiac arrythmias, cardiomyopathy, muscle weakness, elevated triglycerides, mitral valve prolapse, and artherosclerosis.

CoEnzyme Q10 ("CoQ10"), according to the *Physician's Desk Reference*, "is an essential nutrient that is a cofactor in the mitochondrial electron transport chain, the biochemical pathway in cellular respiration from which ATP and metabolic energy is derived. Since nearly all cellular functions are dependent on energy, CoQ10 is essential for the health of all human tissues and organs." (*Physician's Desk Reference*, 1992, p. 2377) Thus, by providing energy to the cell, CoQ10 becomes a powerful antioxidant which protects the body against "free radicals" by neutralizing them before they can cause damage. Free radicals basically "rust" the insides of our bodies causing weakness and cell destruction.

Over 1500 world-wide studies have proven CoQ10's role in preventing (and even curing) all types of heart disease, cancer, periodontal disease, allergies, and high altitude sickness. It is also a powerful energy booster, great for athletes and for those suffering from chronic fatigue syndrome. There are greater deficiencies of this substance in people who limit animal protein as a food source because CoQ10 is found only in animal foods. There may be no better way to slow down the aging process than with the supplementation of CoQ10.

The research literature regarding **ACES** (Vitamins A, C, E, and the mineral Selenium) definitely proves their important role in the protection against "free radical formation," cancer, and heart disease. They all help strengthen the immune system and are powerful anti-aging nutrients. The question is not whether to include ACES in a supplement formula but how to optimize their bioavailability with no side effects. Water dispersion for the fat-soluble vitamin supplements A and E is helpful so that they will be absorbed even if no fat is available. Dry vitamins A and E are beneficial for preventing excess skin oiliness. Recent research has shown that adding a small amount of mixed tocopherol (instead of alpha only) from an oil source enhances the health benefits of Vitamin E. Too much Vitamin E can weaken the immune system so for most individuals, it is best not to exceed 800 i.u. daily.

Vitamin C is critical for human health. Because we are one of the only two animals who cannot manufacture it, we need to supplement this vitamin in our diet. If we had no outside source of Vitamin C, we would get scurvy, which was a common cause of death among the British navy several centuries ago. Excess acid can be caused by taking too much Vitamin C without buffering it with a small amount of calcium carbonate. For optimum bioavailability, it should be taken with bioflavonoids. Quercetin is an excellent, non-allergenic choice.

Selenium is an essential mineral. In parts of the world where selenium is deficient, cancer is far more common. Recent research has proven that with as little as 200 mcg. supplemented daily, selenium offers tremendous protection against several types of cancer. However too much selenium (over 400 mcg. daily on a long term basis) can be toxic.

Because dietary intake and/or absorption of Vitamins A, C, and E and the mineral Selenium may be reduced as humans age, supplementing these in optimum amounts on a daily basis gives people "ACES in the hole" for keeping the immune system healthy and for slowing down the aging process.

4. Liver Detoxifiers:
Lipoic Acid, Glutathione, and Silymarin

Lipoic Acid. Also known as Alpha Lipoic Acid or thioctic acid, is a small, eight-carbon sulfur-containing compound that is essential for energy producing reactions in the body but is not considered a vitamin. Besides being considered a powerful antioxidant (that is both water and fat soluble), improving muscle strength and energy, preventing peripheral neuropathy, chelating heavy metals such as iron and cadmium, and helping regulate blood sugar for diabetes by preventing glycation, lipoic acid is one of the most powerful liver detoxifiers ever discovered. For instance, Burton Berkson, M.D. Ph.D., performed a study in the late 1970's using lipoic acid to stop irreversible liver damage caused by consumption of the amanita mushroom (one of the deadliest poisons in nature). In 100 patients who had sudden liver failure from this and other deadly fungi, over half recovered completely after taking lipoic acid.

Lipoic Acid has a long history of safety; it has been used in Europe for over 30 years with no serious side effects. Toxicity has only been shown in doses over 400-500 mg/kg of body weight.

Glutathione. Technically considered an amino acid, glutathione is a protein produced in the liver from amino acids, cysteine, glutamic acid, and glycine. It helps defend the body against exposure to cigarette smoking, radiation, chemotherapy, and alcohol. It is also a powerful detoxifier of heavy metals and drugs, and aids in the treatment of blood and liver disorders. Because of its ability to neutralize oxygen molecules before they can harm cells, it is a powerful cancer preventive, especially for liver cancer. It also may have an anti-aging benefit.

Silymarin. From the seed of the milk thistle plant, this herb has been used for centuries to treat liver cirrhosis, chronic hepatitis, "fatty" liver, and inflammation of the bile duct. More than 300 clinical and experimental studies have demonstrated its effectiveness.

Silymarin works by slowing the entrance of toxins into liver cells. It also prevents free radical damage and stimulates the production of new liver cells. As individuals age, a healthy liver is crucial for detoxifying additives in foods, medications, and environmental pollutants. If the liver is not operating optimally, fatigue, headaches, and weight gain often ensue. Thus, silymarin is a very safe preventive that can be taken daily. The only side effects may be looser stools for the first few days of use.

5. B-VITAMINS

The water soluble B-complex Vitamins are some of the most studied nutrients and have a wide margin of supplementation safety. They are critical for maintenance of nerve, skin, eye, hair, liver, mouth, and muscle health (including the heart muscle). They also assist digestion and optimize brain function. The B-complex vitamins are coenzymes for the production of energy in the body and are useful in alleviating depression and early Alzheimer's disease. Many of the health problems exhibited by the elderly are directly related to B vitamin deficiencies, either due to improper intake or poor absorption. B vitamins should never be taken alone on a long-term basis because they work as a team and can cause an imbalance if large doses are taken separately.

The most recent research regarding the B vitamins, particularly B-6, B-12, and Folic Acid caused tremendous shock and excitement in the medical community when a recent study reported in the *Journal of the American Medical Association* (*JAMA*, June 1997) that these nutrients may be more important than cholesterol balance in preventing heart disease. In the proper amounts (approximately 75 mg. B-6, 200 mcg. B-12, 800 mcg. Folic Acid) they prevent build-up of plaque in the arteries from hyper homocysteinaemia. Homocysteine is the sulfur-containing by-product of the essential amino acid methionine. Its level can be blood tested. Although this connection was originally discovered by a Harvard Medical School pathologist in 1969, his research was ridiculed while most other medical professionals hopped onto the "cholesterol" bandwagon. Prevention of hyper homocysteinaemia can save millions of lives. Individuals who have a history of heart disease in their family or who already show evidence of high homeocysteine levels should supplement their diets with the proper amounts of B-6, B-12, and folate.

6. Zinc

Zinc. An essential mineral and a catalyst for over 30 bodily functions. Zinc deficiency plays a major role in the following health conditions: acne, anorexia nervosa, delayed sexual maturity, growth impairment, hair loss, fatigue, memory loss; macular degeneration, high LDL cholesterol levels, poor appetite control, impaired night vision, impotence, infertility, acuity of taste and smell, poor protein synthesis, increased susceptibility to infection, skin lesions, propensity for diabetes, prostate enlargement, recurrent colds and flu, and slow wound healing. Major food sources for zinc are fish, shellfish, meat, eggs, soy, and nuts/seeds, especially sunflower seeds. Excess dietary sugar intake depletes zinc stores quickly. Also, compounds in insoluble fibers, particularly whole wheat and psyllium, block zinc's absorption.

Zinc is found in many forms when added to dietary supplements (oxide, aspartate, picolinate, sulphate, chelate, gluconate). Zinc in pill form tends to be absorbed best (with the least side effects if in glycinate/arginate, amino acid, or gluconate bound forms). For warding off colds, flus, and infections, mouth absorption (either gargling with liquid zinc sulfate or sucking zinc lozenges) is essential.

Although supplementing zinc is a must for the aging population or for anyone exhibiting deficiency symptoms, too much supplemental zinc may cause more harm than good. Taking long-term daily doses of over 50 mg. has been shown in some studies to suppress the immune system. The exceptions are illness due to viral or bacterial infections, removal of toxic metal, or recovery from surgery. At these times, it is generally safe to take up to 100 mg. daily on a short-term basis (not for more than two weeks). For individuals concerned about taking too much zinc, a simple screening method is taste-testing with a 10 ml. solution in water. A lack of any taste within a few seconds is an indication of zinc deficiency or poor absorption. This taste test may be particularly helpful to surgical patients because wound healing is mainly enhanced if zinc is proven adequate. Blood serum concentrates are not a good measure of zinc status, but taste testing may be as accurate as a 24 hour urine collection.

Due to the alarming increase in prostate problems among American males over the age of 45, zinc supplementation is critical. The prostate contains a higher percentage of zinc than any other organ in the human body. If this mineral is not maintained at high levels, prostate enlargement and possibly cancerous growths may result.

Retinal zinc deficiency is of particular importance for elderly individuals because it plays a primary role in creating macular degeneration. Low zinc levels may reduce the activity of catalase, an antioxidant enzyme in retinal pigment epithelium, which in turn predisposes to macular degeneration. In addition, zinc deficiency may also impair Vitamin A utilization, which can create many eye problems, including "night blindness."

7. THE ALGAES

Chlorella, Spirulina, and Blue Green Algae are among nature's most ancient food sources. They have been on earth for more than two billion years. They are tiny, single-celled fresh and salt water grown plants that boast one of the best natural sources of protein, vitamins, minerals, chlorophyll, DNA, and RNA. They are complete foods because they contain 19 highly absorbed amino acids and at least twenty vitamins and minerals. Recently, Chlorella, Spirulina, and Blue-Green Algae have been termed "Superfood" nutritional supplements because they are well tolerated and optimally absorbed by most people, even those who have never tolerated nutritional supplements in the past. In most cases, Spirulina contains the highest amount of protein, Chlorella the highest amount of chlorophyll, and Blue Green Algae the most complete food of the three.

Algaes many benefits include: boosting the immune system, aiding digestion, speeding up the healing process, and stimulating optimum metabolism and respiration. Algae supplements are available in powder, liquid, tablet, capsule or tea form. Organic Algae is preferred, because Algae is a harvested, processed plant, and if not organic, could contain unwanted pesticide residue.

8. DIGESTIVE AIDS

Most health experts feel that proper digestion and/or absorption of food is the key to maintaining overall health. Unfortunately, as people age, loss of B-12, digestive enzymes, and hydrochloric acid predisposes them to a variety of preventable health problems. That is why digestive aids are essential for maintenance of optimum health in middle-aged to elderly populations, or in anyone with a compromised digestive system. The most necessary nutrients for optimum digestion are:

B-12. Of all the B-vitamins, probably the most important is B-12 because it aids in cellular energy and is required for proper absorption of foods. Without B-12, it is very difficult to synthesize protein and metabolize carbohydrates and fats.

B-12 deficiencies are very common in the elderly and in anyone suffering from a digestive disorder. This deficiency problem can cause serious symptoms such as abnormal gait, chronic fatigue, constipation, depression, tongue inflammation, irritability, labored breathing, memory loss, moodiness, nervousness, neurological damage, heart palpitations, pernicious anemia, ringing in the ears, and spinal cord degeneration. Because B-12 naturally occurs in only animal foods, all strict vegetarians, people with digestive problems and most people over 45 need to supplement their diets with B-12 to ensure proper absorption of food.

Enzymes. The late Edward Hall, M.D., referred to enzymes as "sparks of life." These energized protein molecules play an important role in all biochemical activities in the human body, including digestion, brain stimulation, cellular energy, and tissue repair. Enzymes are so crucial that even with the perfect balance of vitamins, minerals, water and other nutrients, humans could not survive without them. Naturally occurring enzymes are abundant in raw foods but not in cooked and heavily processed foods. As people age or if they are compromised by poor diets which are enzyme-deficient, enzymes are depleted and may not be able to be replaced. Thus, digestion and absorption of food, even when the diet is healthful, become impaired. By adding digestive enzymes to a dietary supplement formula, absorption of the foods at the meals in which the enzymes are taken will improve dramatically.

Enzymes are secreted along the gastrointestinal tract and break down foods so that the nutrients from those foods may be absorbed into the bloodstream for use in various bodily functions. The three main categories of digestive enzymes are amylase, lipase, and protease.

1. **Amylase**—Amylase is an enzyme found in saliva and pancreatic and intestinal juices. Its main purpose is to digest carbohydrates (complex carbohydrates and simple sugars) in foods. Another carbohydrate metabolizing enzyme is lactase which breaks down milk sugar (lactose). When more than 75% of the world population will become lactose intolerant as they age, lactase is an important supplement addition for most adults who want to consume cow's milk (which is very high in lactose). Maltase is another carbohydrate needed to break down malt sugar (maltose) while sucrase breaks down cane and beet sugars.

2. **Lipase**—Lipase is found primarily in the stomach and pancreatic juices. It is also present in fats occurring naturally in foods and is needed for fat digestion.

3. **Protease.** Protease is found in stomach, pancreatic and intestinal juices. It is essential for protein digestion.

Cellulase. An enzyme used to break down fiber as found in the outer layer of vegetables, fruits, and grains. As humans age, inability to break down these plant fibers may cause abdominal distress, including gas and bloating.

Because the ability to produce digestive enzymes decreases as we age, it is vital for elderly people to enhance nutrient absorption. It is also beneficial for everyone to include naturally occurring enzymes in their diet, particularly from foods such as avocado, papaya, pineapple, banana, mango, and sprouts.

Probiotics. These are healthful bacteria (i.e. Bifidobacterium, Lactobacillus, Streptococcus, Enterococcus) that prevent or reduce the effect of pathogenic organisms that invade the body through the digestive tract. The human gastrointestinal (GI) tract is a bacterium's paradise. Bacteria that produce lactic acid, such as probiotics, suppress the growth of pathogens while having little effect on healthful bacteria. When too little lactic acid is present in the GI tract, pathogens multiply, thus setting the stage for infection, disease, malabsorption of nutrients, and prevention of B-vitamin synthesis. According to Dr. Khem Shahani, P.h.D., worldwide authority of GI microorganisms for over 30 years and author of over 200 scientific papers on the topic, "it is of essence to human health that a probiotic internal environment be established."

Thus, an active culture of probiotics, especially *Lactobacillus acidophilus* taken in an active yogurt or viable supplement form can prevent or minimize lactose intolerance, foodborne illnesses, and restore bowel function that has been compromised by poor diet or yeast imbalance.

Hydrochloric Acid. As people age, they produce less hydrochloric acid (HCL). HCL is an essential substance for digesting protein from foods. Also, with America's obsession for turning off stomach acid through the overuse of antacids such as TUMS®, Tagamet®, and Zantac®, hypochlorhydria (low stomach acid) or achlorhydria (no stomach acid) can occur. Without stomach acid, hard-to-digest foods are so poorly absorbed that diarrhea and/or undigested food particles will appear. Also it is rather ironic that TUMS® are recommended as a calcium source to prevent Osteoporosis when it is known that the calcium carbonate in TUMS® alkalizes stomach acid which is needed to absorb calcium. If calcium cannot be absorbed, urinary calcium excretion increases or worse, calcium deposits may form in breast, bone, joint, or kidney tissue causing problems such as kidney stones and heel/bone spurs.

Supplementation of a small amount of hydrochloric acid in a vitamin/mineral formula (Betaine HCL) that also has added B-12, B-6, and Zinc to stimulate our digestive tract into making HCL, is very helpful for optimizing nutrient absorption from food.

9. GINKGO BILOBA

Ginkgo Biloba. A standardized leaf extract (GBE), taken in supplement form in a capsule or tincture, has a low level of toxicity and has been well-researched for providing a wide variety of health benefits. The Ginkgo tree from which the leaf extract is taken has been virtually unchanged for 150 million years!

The Chinese have used Ginkgo for thousands of years to treat various health conditions such as asthma, allergies, and coughs; and in the West it is now among the most popular herbal remedies for use as an energizer, mood lifter, and as a "smart drug." Ginkgo has been shown to increase brain function, memory, alertness, and antioxidation.

For allergy, inflammation and asthma prevention, gingko works by disarming platelet activating factors (PAF), key chemical causes of these conditions. Ginkgo molecules known as ginkgolides, compete with PAF for binding sites, thus inhibiting the inflammation, smooth muscle contraction and bronchoconstriction.

With regards to treating cerebrovascular disease, more than 40 double-blind studies have shown its effectiveness. In fact, Ginkgo Biloba extract (GBE) is a registered drug in Germany and France and is among the leading prescriptions for treating cerebrovascular disease in these two countries in a dosage of 40 mg. three times daily.

Ginkgo Biloba is now being researched for delaying mental deterioration among Alzheimer's patients and has shown promising preliminary results. For dementia due to vascular insufficiency or dementia not related to Alzheimer's, GBE will usually improve mental function in a standardized dosage of 40 mg. three times daily. In fact, in a recent study of patients suffering from senile dementia, significant improvements in memory and attention were witnessed among those individuals who took GBE in the standardized dosage.

For treating peripheral vascular insufficiency, clinical trials measuring GBE have been found effective in inhibiting platelet aggregation, improving blood flow to ischemic areas, increasing walking distance, enhancing energy production, and reducing pain at rest.

More research is needed for GBE's use among the younger generation who swear by it as a "smart drug." College students in large numbers have taken to this ancient herb because they have found it enhances memory and alertness better than many drugs. Its benefits over drugs are few side effects, low cost, and availability without prescription. As research continues to escalate, there is no question that there will be more recommended uses for Ginkgo Biloba. Otherwise, why would the tree have survived for 150 million years?

10. SAW PALMETTO (FOR MALES ONLY)

An estimated one-half of all American males over 50 have problems with enlargement of the prostate gland which wreaks havoc on the bladder. This condition is known as benign prostatic hypertrophy (BPH). Also, cancer of the prostate is occurring at an alarming rate among American males. To the rescue comes **Saw Palmetto**, an extract of the berries from a palm tree native to the Southern Atlantic coast that has been used for centuries to nourish prostate, as an aphrodisiac and to assist the male reproductive system.

Over 20 double-blind, placebo controlled studies have demonstrated that this fat-soluble extract of saw palmetto berries is very effective in eliminating the major symptoms of BPH; in fact, even more effective than Proscar, the prescription drug used to medically treat BPH (*The American Journal of Natural Medicine*, September 1994), and has far fewer, if any, side effects. Although there has been no direct evidence linking Saw Palmetto to prostate cancer prevention, it is known that the majority of men suffering from untreated BPH will go on to develop cancer. Thus, reducing the size of the prostate gland with Saw Palmetto and adding the mineral, zinc, to nourish the prostate gland are certainly worthwhile recommendations for keeping the prostate as healthy as possible.

Personal Case Study #7

I have never seen such dramatic health improvements as among magnesium deficient individuals when they add it as a supplement to their diets. Sam B. is a professional golfer who was overweight, fatigued and popped pain relievers like candy due to severe muscle exertion pain. His fiancee begged him to seek nutritional advice.

Besides consuming diet soda and fast food, he drank at least a six-pack of beer every time he partied with his golfing friends. He told me that he honestly did not know if he was willing to make the dietary changes that I suggested.

Within three days of taking large doses of Magnesium Gylcinate, his muscle pain disappeared and what he defined as "mild depression for no reason" lifted. He said that he then found it easy to eliminate all diet sodas (which depletes magnesium) and to cut back on beer intake. The unexpected bonus was eloping with his fiancee on St. Patrick's Day. It also did not hurt that the "tire" around his belly melted away and his concentration during golf tournaments improved.

❈ 8 ❊

Free Food Choices...
Who Said Nothing in Life is Free?

How many things in life are really free? Fortunately, many food substances are nutritious, satisfying, and virtually calorie free so that they can be enjoyed in moderation. In this chapter, we will highlight several of the most common "free foods" which go beyond mere sustenance and providing fuel; they envelop the senses with aromas and delicious flavors of food that make eating pleasurable.

HERBS AND SPICES

Before they were used for seasonings, culinary herbs and spices were most likely used for food preservation. In particular, antimicrobial activity (to kill bacteria, fungi, parasites, and viruses) in the most potent amounts are found in raw and minimally processed garlic, onion, turmeric, ginger, sage, rosemary, oregano, and cayenne pepper.

Herbs, synonymous with vegetables in ancient times, also have medicinal value. Many have actually been ingredients in making many commonly used medications. For instance, white willow bark is the major ingredient in aspirin. Table I highlights some of the most ancient herbs and their uses.

Plant foods, but particularly fruits and vegetables (including herbs), were referred to in biblical passages constantly for their medicinal and healing properties. For instance, in Ezekiel 47:12, it is said, *And on the banks, on both sides of the river, there will grow all kinds of trees for food. Their leaves will not wither nor their fruit fail, but they will bear fresh fruit every month, because the water for them flows from the sanctuary. Their fruit will be for food and their* **leaves for healing**. For instance, the molasses made from pomegranate is not only great tasting but is also a powerful medicine. An infusion from the root of the pomegranate was used in ancient times to rid the body of tapeworm infestations.

PLANT POWER

Today science is proving what ancient man already knew . . . that fruits and vegetables contain fantastic healing properties. The phytochemicals in plant foods that have been most extensively researched have been the allicin in garlic, the large amounts of beta carotene found in orange, yellow, and red-colored fruits and vegetables, indoles found in cruciferous vegetables (i.e. broccoli, cauliflower, cabbage, brussel sprouts), and genistein and phytoestrogens found in soybeans. Preliminary evidence indicates that allicin, beta carotene, indoles, and genistein can prevent and assist in curing various forms of cancer, help stimulate the immune system, and slow the growth of degenerative diseases.

LOW STARCH VEGETABLES

The unhealthiest people in the world rarely, if ever, eat vegetables. Low starch vegetable choices can actually be enjoyed in an unlimited amount for most people because they are complex carbohydrates that are low in calories, contain no fat, may be high in fiber, and have powerful disease-fighting properties. Some of the best low starch vegetables include greens, kale, kelp, leeks, onions, garlic, seaweed, and sprouts (especially onion and broccoli sprouts).

THE SALT OF THE EARTH

Of all the herbs and spices, salt has been the most popular and useful throughout history. Scientifically, we know that humans would die without sodium (table salt is sodium chloride). Salt acts as a stimulant to the adrenals and elevates blood pressure, which can lead to a better mental state and a feeling of warmth and alertness. Salt is also an inexpensive, effective preservative. In ancient times, its use in preservation of animal foods was detailed in the Kosher dietary laws, which are still adhered to in many cultures today.

If salt is so essential to life, why does it have such a negative image today? The pure and simple answers are overuse and adding harmful additives to sodium. The average human needs between 1,100 and 3,300 mg. of sodium per day for optimum cell function. Most Americans consume between 4,000 and 10,000 mg. daily. Only one teaspoon of table salt contains about 2,000 mg. of sodium. But most of the sodium overload in the U.S. comes from hidden sodium compounds (nitrates, caseinates, benzoates, and monosodium glutamate) found in overly processed food. These components have been linked to hypertension (high blood pressure), edema, and strokes and should be avoided completely. Moderation in all things is the way to live. The use of sodium from natural sources, such as sea salt, is just one more example of this concept.

TEA . . . THE CIVILIZED DRINK

Extracts of fruits, herbs, and vegetables have been used for at least 4,000 years in soothing, health-building medicinal teas. To the ancient Greeks tea was the "divine leaf" and used for asthma, colds and bronchitis. Many of the extracts made into tea (see Table I) have been historically used to destroy bacteria and viruses, fight infections, lower blood pressure, soothe the "weary soul," and retard atherosclerosis (hardening of the arteries). Recent research has proven the cancer preventing and fighting properties of certain teas, especially black and green. Prominent cancer researcher, John Weisburger, drinks about five cups of tea each day and says this amount of tea delivers as much antioxidant benefit as two fruits or vegetables. Several cautions with tea: too much may block iron absorption so more than two cups daily are not recommended for anemic individuals and pregnant women. (Pregnant women should consult with a nutritionist or health care professional before consuming herb teas, since certain herbs may actually be harmful to the baby.) Tea can stimulate gastric acid so is not recommended for ulcer sufferers; the caffeine found in most teas may be too stimulating for some individuals (especially for children). Excess tea consumption may wear down the enamel on your teeth. An optimum amount for most adults is two cups of strong tea daily.

COFFEE

Scholars aren't sure that coffee as we know it today is the same kind of coffee that was consumed in ancient times. We do know, however, that today's dark brown drink made from roasted and ground seeds of the tropical coffee plant has been a dietary staple and medicine for at least the last few centuries. The caffeine in coffee has the benefits of giving you a mental lift, "jump-starting" your brain for better performance on mental tasks, reducing wheezing and asthma symptoms by opening bronchial passages, and providing a spurt of energy to athletes. The down-side is that coffee can be addictive; it can induce or aggravate headaches, insomnia, anxiety, heartburn, and heart palpitations; it can raise blood cholesterol levels; it can cause problems to the fetuses of pregnant women; it may encourage osteoporosis by depleting calcium and magnesium; and because it is very irritating to the bladder.

Moderation is the key when it comes to coffee consumption. One or two cups each day should pose no health risks for most adults. If symptoms arise, it is best to stop drinking coffee entirely. Decaffeinated coffee may be an acceptable alternative, but is higher in acid than most caffeinated coffees. Also, unless it is water-processed, decaf coffee could contain residues of the dangerous chemical, methylene chloride.

Cereal grain coffees, such as Postum, Pero, Roma, or Bambuu are a satisfying drink choice for those of us who don't want or can't drink coffee. Strong barley tea is also a good coffee substitute because it aids digestion and tastes and smells a lot like the real thing. Cereal grain coffees should be avoided by anyone suffering from grain allergies.

What a Lemon!

One of the best detoxifiers and digestive aids for most people is the fresh lemon. Lemon in sparkling or plain water is a refreshing non-caloric drink that has medicinal value. Eating the inside of a lemon rind is also highly recommended because that is where the powerful bioflavonoids are concentrated to strengthen the immune system and protect the integrity of artery walls. So the next time someone says that "you got a real lemon" . . . thank them!

Personal Case Study #8

One of my most difficult challenges as a nutrition counselor is restricting portions for weight loss purposes. Many people become despondent when they have to count their proteins, carbos and fats. That's why it is such a pleasure to allow an unlimited intake of low starch vegetables, herbal teas and aromatic spices.

Harold J. was a coffee taster who had never been able to stick to a weight loss diet for more than three weeks because diet foods were too bland, and when dieting, his taste buds diminished so much that it interfered with his job.

Besides making sure his zinc level was normal (zinc deficiency affects taste and smell dramatically), we planned menus using a wide array of aromatic greens, herbs and spices. He has been able to stick to his newly designed Food Plan (I never use the term diet) for the last two years with only slight modifications. He cannot believe that he never feels deprived. His new interest in using a wide variety of herbs and spices has even helped him develop new coffee blends, using aromatic spices instead of cream, and natural sweeteners for enhanced flavor.

TABLE I
HERBS FOR FOOD AND MEDICINAL USE

HERB	HISTORY	USE	CAUTIONS	Medicinal Properties
Cinnamon		• great spice for breads, cakes, muffins, pancakes Sticks are also great in cider.	• in heavy concentrations, may be irritating to the skin & mucus membrane in the mouth • if salicylate sensitive, may cause an allergic reaction	• may relieve upset stomach, gas, and diarrhea (2–5 drops of the oil in warm water)
Cloves	This dried bud of the clove tree was used regularly in China for more than 2000 yrs. & legend described it as an aphrodisiac.	• spice for Eastern Med. dishes, breads, muffins & pies.		• old remedy for footaches • antiseptic properties • to relieve regurgitation (2–5 drops of oil in cup of water)
Cucumber	Since ancient times, cucumber juice has been used as a facial cleanser & treatment for skin irritation. Cleopatra was reputed to have used this to preserve her skin.	• great for soups & salads	• hard to digest esp. with the skin left on, so may cause stomachaches	• good diuretic & can help prevent constipation • may bring down high blood cholesterol levels • cucumber slices on the eyes may reduce swelling • relieves sunburn & other skin irritations
Garlic (Onion has similar properties, but is less potent)	Ancient Egyptians worshipped garlic & fed it to their slaves to keep them healthy. Hippocrates even used it in 460 B.C. to treat uterine cancer.	• pungent aroma makes any main dish, veg. or grain dish taste fabulous	• overuse can cause digestive imbalance • overuse can cause body odor • topical use may cause redness & swelling to an infected area	• research has shown this to be the wonder drug of the world because it has natural immune boosting properties • reduces high blood pressure & cholesterol levels • used as a cancer preventive

	Benefits	Cautions	Uses
Garlic (continued)	• kills bacteria & other troublesome microorganism • treats ear, yeast, skin & other infections • anticoagulent • excellent digestive aid	• don't eat more than 10 cloves per day – it can be toxic or trigger allergies; also large amounts of garlic eaten by lactating women can cause colic in their infant	
Horseradish	• good expectorant • diuretic, aids digestion • soothes respiratory tract • may relieve asthma symptoms & coughs • stimulates blood flow to inflamed joints	• so bitter if eaten alone that it can bring tears to the eyes	• used externally–to relieve pain & stiffness of rheumatism • used sparingly to flavor mustards & other condiments
Mint (Peppermint)	• tea soothes headaches, possibly even migraines • tea aids digestion • if you have too little stomach acid, peppermint may relieve heartburn or gas • may soothe mild cough	• don't use if your digestive tive tract is too acidic • don't use if salicylate sensitive	• great as a tea & in candies & gum
Olive	• leaves may reduce fevers & is a mild tranquilizer • oil reduces "bad" LDL chol & raises "good" HDL chol • may prevent heart disease • stimulates production of bile in the liver • gentle laxative relieves constipation (drink 1-2 oz. in the morning) • can soothe insect bites, itching, dry skin & bruises • good hair conditioner for dry scalp	• do not use a large amount of the oil as a laxative during pregnancy	• the fruit is a wonderful addition to salads, & grain dishes • olives are also wonderful eaten alone. Olive oil is very flavorful for salads & all Mediterranean dishes.

On the seder, the traditional Passover meal today commemorates the suffering of the Jews under Pharoah's rule. (Horseradish)

Since biblical times the branch of an olive tree has been a symbol of peace & prosperity. The entire plant is useful. (Olive)

TABLE I (*continued*)
HERBS FOR FOOD AND MEDICINAL USE

HERB	HISTORY	USE	CAUTIONS	Medicinal Properties
Parsley		• all soups, main dishes & grain dishes to add color & flavor • makes a wonderful tea to aid digestion & to freshen breath after eating garlic	• pregnant women should not take parsley juice or oil (too potent) • helps congestion due to coughs and colds • soothing for asthma • oil may induce menstrat. • cancer preventive • diuretic good for reduction of fluid retention (edema)	• relieves gas • aids digestion & settles stomach after a meal
Senna		• aids elimination in pill or tea forms	• consistent usage may cause dependency	• reverses constipation • strong laxative

❧ 9 ❧

Feel Great, Look Great

PREVENTION OF ILLNESS AND DEGENERATIVE DISEASE
THROUGH A HEALTHY LIFESTYLE AND DIET

More nutrition research has been performed in the last five years than throughout history. Nutrition research has proven that the optimum diet for good health is the same diet that was eaten and recommended for thousands of years. According to S. Boyd Eaton, M.D., of Emory University in Atlanta, Georgia, anthropologist Melvin Konner, and a growing number of physicians and nutritionists, ancient diets are genetically what we are designed to eat, digest, and metabolize. Veering too far from this nutritional program is one of the main reasons why modern humans so often suffer from "diseases of civilization," which include cancer, hypertension, heart disease, and diabetes. These "diseases of civilization" are among the top killers in Western Society but are virtually unknown among the few surviving hunter-gatherer and nomadic populations. For example, when diabetic Australian Aborigines living near Melbourne returned to their hunter-gatherer lifestyle, their diabetic abnormalities disappeared (*Diabetes*, June, 1984).

How drastically has the diet of Western societies changed in the last 50 years? According to research of ancient cultures, our diets have changed more in the last 50 years than throughout history. Many of the "foods" eaten today are man-made, which has given humans very little time to make the genetic changes that are necessary to tolerate them. A recent survey of the most-purchased supermarket items (*Washington Post*, December, 1992) reported Coca-Cola, Pepsi-Cola, Diet Pepsi, and Diet Coca-Cola as the big winners. All four of these are "chemicals in a can." The next most popular items were canned soup, canned tomato paste, canned tuna, boxed macaroni and cheese, and boxed corn bread mix. These popular items, except for the tuna and tomato paste, are usually over-processed, chemical-laden, nutrient-poor items that bear little resemblance to their natural counterparts. Where were the fresh fruits, vegetables, legumes, and whole grains on this list? If these whole foods had been the most frequently purchased items, the degenerative disease rate in the Western world would be rapidly declining instead of uncontrollably rising

THE BEST AND WORST FOODS FOR BUILDING HEALTH

Based upon the most up-to-date scientific research, the following foods are the WORST because they contribute to weight gain and degenerative disease.

1. **Soft drinks.** This is the epitome of nutritional bankruptcy. Diet sodas are the worst . . . addictive and in large amounts, neurotoxic. If you're desperate for something sweet and fizzy, have fruit juice mixed with sparkling mineral water.

2. **French fries.** These are the "black eyes" of the potato. A baked potato is nutrient-dense, high in complex carbohydrates, and low in calories. When you fry them in beef or hydrogenated vegetable fats, they acquire another 200 calories of sludge that we expect our gastrointestinal tracts to digest.

3. **Potato chips.** And you thought French Fries were a health disaster? You might as well eat straight butter, which is probably better for you in the long run because most potato chips are fried in unnatural, hydrogenated fat.

4. **Bacon.** This is not really meat; it is saturated meat fat. As many as 95% of the calories in bacon come from fat. Bacon is also high in sodium, and the chemical nitrates

that are released from frying this grease can cause cancers of the digestive tract.

5. **Fast food "superburgers"** Most of these "wonders of chemistry" contain 500–600 calories, and at least one-half of these calories come from fat, not to mention the added sodium that provides more than your daily ration. Also, their questionable preparation and handling practices make these burgers a playground for salmonella, E. coli, and other pathogens. Eating a "superburger" is like playing a game of Russian roulette with your good health.

6. **Doughnuts.** This is worse than no food at all. Not only do doughnuts contain too much sugar and bleached white flour, but they're also fried in grease. When eaten for breakfast, they put your blood sugar out-of-whack, sit like a brick in your stomach, and don't even give you the stamina to keep going until lunch.

7. **"Those cute little cupcakes made by the big food giants"** Don't believe them when they tell you that the shelf-life of these pseudo-foods is only a few days. It is a known fact that they can last forever . . . they become fossilized but are never touched by mold or bacteria. They provide a large number of calories, big doses of fat and sugar, and a list of chemical additives that even a biochemist can't translate. If even mold and bacteria won't feed upon them, why do we?

8. **Artificial snack foods.** These "goodies" from the food and chemical giants' arsenal enter the American marketplace to the tune of 20 new items weekly. We can choose from fake corn chips, fake potato chips (as if the real thing isn't bad enough), fake fruits as recommended by superstars, granola bars (that you are fooled into thinking are healthy), and cereals that are more harmful than eating candy. If you want to destroy your health while putting a fortune into the food giants' pockets, these are the treats for you.

Isn't it ironic that all of the **BEST** foods, as determined by scientific research, have been consumed the longest? They are as follows:

1. **Vegetables.** All fresh or plain frozen vegetables are highly recommended. You really can't eat too many of these. They are all good sources of fiber and complex carbohydrates. Many are very low in calories. Some of the healthiest choices include onions, garlic, carrots, broccoli, cabbage, brussels sprouts, sweet potatoes, and squash.

2. **Fruits.** Nature's bounties of sweetness are pleasing to the palate while providing important nutrients. Some of the super fruits include melons, olives (from which olive oil is made), avocados (they're high in potassium, B-6, and magnesium and their fat is monounsaturated), bananas, kiwi, and papaya.

3. **Whole grains.** Whole grain foods are staples for every country in the world. Their fiber and nutrients are "life-giving," and there is virtually no fat to be found in whole grains except for a trace of Vitamin E oil. Whole Wheat and wheat germ should be kept to a minimum because large amounts block mineral absorption. Wheat intolerance is also a very common problem worldwide.

4. **Legumes.** Dried peas, lentils, garbanzos and other beans are excellent sources of vegetable protein and fiber, aid digestion, regulate blood serum cholesterol levels, and are some of the least expensive foods to buy and the easiest to prepare. The **peanut** is a legume to be eaten with caution because it is a common allergen and often contains an aflatoxin mold.

5. **Fish.** Fish is not only tasty, but nutritious as well. Modern scientific research has proclaimed fish to be an excellent source of protein. It has also proven the omega-3 fatty acids found in fish (especially salmon, mackerel, and sardines) to be heart healthy. To varying degrees, different types of fish protect against blood clots and cancer

while stimulating the immune system. Fish is a rich source of the mineral, zinc, which is critical for growth, sexual function, good eyesight, appetite control, absorption of carbohydrates and protein, and a healthy immune system. And if these facts aren't enough, fish is also low in calories which can benefit any weight loss diet. Be sure that your fish comes from safe waters (see Chapter 4 for details). (Adapted from *Center for Science in the Public Interest Newsletter*)

MAINTAINING OPTIMUM WEIGHT

Weight loss is big business world-wide, but especially in the United States where one out of every three Americans is certifiably overweight. The most alarming aspect of obesity in America is that the proportion of American children who are overweight has increased more than 50 percent over the last two decades. In 1990 alone, Americans spent an estimated $35 billion for diet books, diet soft drinks, appetite suppressants, group weight loss programs and liquid diet supplements. Most people are willing to try anything for the chance of becoming thinner. Has all of this time and money brought good results? Slim chance . . . at any given time, at least one-half of the American population is on a weight loss diet and 95 percent of them will not only regain all their lost weight, but will add excess weight from fat. So every time a dieter goes on a weight loss diet, there is less of a chance to lose weight and regain good health.

Severely reduced calorie diets don't work, even though weight appears to drop off initially at a substantial rate. But instead of losing fat, what's really accounting for the quick weight loss is consumption of the body's temporary energy reserve, in the form of glycogen, and its associated water. As hunger inevitably returns, the glycogen and water also return (which is why many people seem to reach a plateau in their weight loss attempts). The fat stores remain virtually untouched. Any diet that promises a weight loss of more than one or two pounds per week is either counting on this very temporary weight loss or is a very calorie-restricted diet, which puts the body into starvation mode. When a diet supplies too few calories to support the basal metabolic rate, the body will hold on to precious fat molecules for what it perceives as famine times ahead and switches to lean muscle tissue for fuel. Consequently, the body's metabolic rate will slow down to conserve energy for its new "survival mode."

Restricted food intake also prevents adequate nutrient intake, unless vitamin and mineral supplements are taken, protein is adequate, and enough calories are consumed to meet individual energy needs. To meet energy needs, the average moderately-active adult female needs a minimum of 1200 calories per day while the average man needs at least 1600 calories per day.

If a dieter has employed a severely restricted food intake regimen, the weight gain when normal food intake occurs will be dramatic. In the dieter's former "starvation mode metabolism," fat absorption becomes so efficient that the inevitable weight gain will be in "fat" instead of in "muscle" pounds. According to obesity researcher, Kelly Brownell, PhD. of the University of Pennsylvania School of Medicine, *it's as though dieting teaches the body a lesson. An organism that is repeatedly deprived of food increases its chances of survival if it learns to store food more efficiently when it is available. When food is once again scarce, the body shuts down its calorie-burning furnace.* Obviously, severely restricting food intake is not the scientifically recommended method for losing weight.

THE TEN COMMANDMENTS FOR LOSING WEIGHT

If gluttony, starvation, and restricted weight loss diets are inappropriate methods for maintaining optimum health and weight, what are the best ways to achieve total balance? The following Ten Commandments for Losing Weight, based on the latest scientific evidence, can be easily achieved with minimal effort. So, what are you waiting for . . . go for it!

I. Do not overeat.

II. Eat enough calories to meet **energy needs** (usually 1200 per day for a moderately active woman and 1600 per day for a moderately active man).

III. Eat enough calories to provide **adequate nutrient intake** (it usually is impossible for a growing teenager or adult to consume adequate protein, vitamins, minerals, carbohydrates, and fats on a diet of less than 1000 calories per day).

IV. Eat at least three meals daily or five mini-meals to regulate blood sugar and to prevent hunger.

V. Don't diet ... instead, adopt a healthy eating plan at any stage in life and mix it with a healthy dose of activity to shed extra pounds and to achieve safe, lasting results.

VI. Eat a wide variety of foods, from the "Best" Choices listed in your Food Plan. (See Appendix A).

VII. Avoid foods that are not well digested or that cause allergy/sensitivity reactions (our bodies can't build muscle and burn fat if we're out-of-balance).

VIII. Eat real food (our bodies can't effectively process or remove "fake food" ingredients without causing us to lose valuable nutrients).

IX. Give your digestive tract a chance to rest with a 24-hour fast at least once every six months (except for infants, young children, and those who are medically impaired).

X. Optimize your lifestyle (reduce stress, avoid tobacco, avoid drugs and prescribed medications unless absolutely necessary, drink in moderation—if at all, drink enough "safe" water, exercise, and **smell the roses!**).

Personal Case Study #9

Vanessa L. was a 53 year old housekeeper who was only paid for the days she worked. Since her total hysterectomy three years earlier she had gained 35 pounds, was always fatigued and had such severe arthritic symptoms and edema (fluid retention) that she couldn't work more than two days per week, and only then if she took NSAIDs daily, which gave her a stomachache. Just recently she had developed itching and occasional hives. She popped buffered aspirin constantly which only seemed to make her worse.

After reviewing her health history, food diary and pill intake, it was clear that Vanessa produced excess acid and fluid. Premarin, an estrogen prescribed for menopausal symptoms, aspirin (salicylic acid) prescribed for pain, 2,000 milligrams of Vitamin C (ascorbic acid) and her diet appeared to be the main culprits. Her diet consisted mainly of fatty pork and beef, corn, tomatoes, peppers and white potatoes. She used too much salt, cayenne, white and black pepper as seasonings.

Vanessa and I had to plan her nutrition program in stages. First, we eliminated the ascorbic acid (switched to Sago Palm Vitamin C), stopped the aspirin (switched to non-aspirin) and stopped all intake of tomatoes, peppers and potatoes (nightshade plants). Her spices of choice were changed to parsley, fresh lemon, garlic and onions. Olive oil was added to substitute for the lard and margarine in her diet. Magnesium was added for acid balance, better muscle metabolism, and pain relief.

Vanessa saw a dramatic improvement in her arthritis, pain, itching, hives within one month of making the changes, but still suffered from fluid retention, exhaustion and had not lost weight. Our next step was to add B-Vitamins, especially B-6, which reduces fluid retention and zinc in the form of fish, nuts and seeds. A liquid zinc and water drink was added for better absorption, weight loss and healing. We also contacted her gynecologist who agreed to switch her from oral Premarin (which is processed by the liver) to a skin absorbed estrogen patch.

Two weeks later Vanessa stopped by my office on her way to work reporting an energy level that she had not felt since she was 20. She wanted to use my scale to be sure that she actually lost 12 pounds. I explained that she had removed a huge amount of excess fluid and now we would be hoping for a one and one-half to two pound consistent weekly weight loss. She said she no longer needed her pain and arthritis medications as long as she avoided nightshade plants and fatty meats.

Two years later Vanessa came in for a nutritional fine-tuning. She appeared happier and more radiant than either of us could have imagined. She told me that her increased energy and pain-free living had given her the courage to start her own housekeeping service that was becoming quite successful. She had two employees and no longer had to perform housework herself, but still wanted to put in a hard day's work just to make sure she could still do it, pain-free. With her svelte figure (5´7, 140 pounds), I had no doubt she could run circles around the rest of her employees. Vanessa was also proud to tell me that her employees used only environmentally friend-ly cleaning supplies because she now realized that many of the toxic chemicals that she used to breathe in daily had contributed to the muscle pain and fatigue.

℘ 10 ℘

It's All in the Genes

According to Dr. Artemis Simopoulos, head of The Center for Genetics, Nutrition, and Health in Washington, D.C., "the interaction of genetics and environment, nature and nurture, is the foundation for all health and disease." Specifically with regards to the optimum diet for humans, nuclear DNA mutations have accounted for a miniscule 0.005% change in our genetic structure. Thus, our genes today are very similar to those of man during the Paleolithic period of 40,000 years ago. During the Paleolithic period, humans consumed more protein, calcium (from bones, not dairy foods), potassium, ascorbic acid, and omega 3 fatty acids than do most humans living today. Even though there is extensive research evidence that genetic variation and differences in gene-nutrient interactions exist among individuals, most Western countries have chosen to adopt a one-size fits all approach to dietary recommendations to prevent or treat degenerative diseases. This approach, as in The U.S.D.A. Food Pyramid, does not work. It does not pay attention to individual differences, nor does it recommend different disease prevention diets.

To date, our easiest approach to understanding our individual genetic code is through knowledge of our Blood Type. Understanding our Blood Type also assists our understanding of how much our DNA has evolved in the last 40,000 years. Blood typing originated with the pioneering work of Karl Landsteiner, M.D. in the early 1900s. Collectively, the four main blood types (O, A, B, and AB) became known as ABO blood groups. Researchers discovered that ABO blood groups were genetically transmitted from parents to their children. Although most of

121

us are familiar with the standard ABO blood typing system, few of us realize how important our blood type is as a clue to which lifestyle system and dietary plan is best for us. Eating the optimum foods for our genetic code (blood type) optimizes our digestion and absorption of those foods while reducing our risk for various diseases.

Peter D'Adamo (*Eat Right for your Type*, 1996) and his predecessors (especially his father, J. D'Adamo, and Toshitaka Nomi et al.) popularized our understanding of how our genetic memory passed on to us through our ancestors affects us physically, mentally, and emotionally. They performed research showing that individuals with a specific blood type react to specific foods because of an imbalance between the molecules in the food and the cell surface antigens of the digestive tract present in various blood groups. This incompatibility leads to the body's "fighting itself," resulting in the increased risk for various diseases. Following is a brief description of the four main blood types and how they may relate to an optimum diet and lifestyle:

O — This is the most ancient blood type, our true paleolithic ancestors of 40,000 years ago. Blood type Os have the genetic needs of hunter-gatherers, have the shortest intestinal tract, and should be carnivores (meat eaters). They absorb vegetable protein very poorly so should never be Vegans (avoiding all animal protein sources). They digest domesticated grains poorly but thrive on ancient wild grasses (such as quinoa). They do not tolerate most cow's milk products. Their most absorbable calcium is derived from ground bone. Blood Type Os thrive on lean animal protein, fatty fish, most nuts/seeds, root vegetables, most fruits, and wild grasses. Blood Type Os typically feel best if their diet contains at least 60% protein and healthy fats. They also thrive on strenuous physical activity.

Blood type O Negative is the universal donor (can give blood to all other blood types) but can only receive blood from another "O." Blood type O makes up about 45% of the world's population.

A — This blood type evolved in Asia or the Middle East between 15,000 and 25,000 B.C. when the environment changed drastically. These Neolithic people developed a more domesticated agrarian lifestyle, stable communities, and permanent living structures. Neolithic people developed mutations of the intestinal tract (a longer length being a presumed part of this), allowing them to tolerate and absorb cultivated products better. Type As are less prone to infectious diseases, but are very sensitive to chemical food additives and pesticides. They have weak digestive enzymes for digesting heavy meats and whole wheat. They also become lactose intolerant after childhood so cannot tolerate cow's milk as adults. They typically do well with fermented dairy products (such as cheese and yogurt). Some type As can be "adaptive vegetarians" if they consume enough vegetable and animal by-product proteins (such as eggs and fermented dairy products) on a consistent basis. There is no proof that ancient blood type As were strictly vegetarian. Even if they couldn't find fish or freshly killed animals, they were known to eat snakes and insects for nourishment (good protein sources). Type As do not thrive on strenuous exercise; they feel much better with endurance exercises (i.e. long walks or hikes instead of short runs).

Blood type A can receive blood from A and O and can give blood to A and AB. Blood type A makes up about 40% of the world's population today.

B — This blood type developed between 10,000 and 15,000 B.C. in the Himalayan highlands, and may have initially mutated in response to climactic changes among a mix of Caucasian and Mongolian tribes. Blood type Bs were originally a nomadic population, eventually migrating to Europe, Asia, and the Americas. Blood Type Bs do best on a well-balanced, varied diet. They tolerate most animal protein well, including milk products from domesticated animals. Most type Bs cannot tolerate whole wheat, corn, and buckwheat. Because they are prone to viral infections, they do not tolerate chicken well. In my practice, I have seen many milk sensitivities among Blood type Bs. This appears to be due to the fact that American cattle are fed large amounts of corn. Typically, when Bs consume milk products from non-corn fed animals, they digest milk well. Type Bs do best with balance in all areas of their lives and do not accept major changes easily. From an exercise standpoint, they thrive with a combination of strenuous exercise (i.e. aerobics, running) and mind-body activities (i.e. yoga or tai chi).

Blood type B can receive blood from B or O, but can only give to B and AB. Blood type B makes us about 10% of the world's population today.

AB — Because this blood type emerged only between 1,000 and 1,200 years ago, it is the rarest. An intermingling of Type A Caucasians with Type B Mongolians created this blood type when a large western migration of eastern peoples took place 10–12 centuries ago. Blood type ABs appear to have the healthiest immune systems because they have an enhanced ability to manufacture more specific antibodies to microbial infections. They also appear to be able to tolerate the most foods because their digestive mutations had over 38,000 years to evolve. Type ABs thrive on a diet that combines the best choices of Blood Type A and B. Their best exercise regimen combines endurance, strenuous, and mind-body activities.

Blood type AB is the universal receiver (can receive blood from all but can only give blood to another AB). Blood type AB makes up about 5% of the world's population today.

The fascinating dietary information gleaned from relating blood types to food intake brings further proof that optimal eating is based on individual needs. I have even noticed in clinical practice that individuals who have parents with different blood types should adapt their own diets to approximately 60–70% of the diet for their blood type and 30–40% from their parents' blood types, if different from their own. One diet clearly does not fit all just as one size shoe does not fit all.

Your Personal Food Plan (see Appendix A) incorporates blood type information, along with research regarding the health benefits of non-toxic, nutrient-dense food choices. Portions of proteins, carbohydrates, and fats should always be in balance and based on energy expenditure and lifestyle factors.

Prologue

Just as the medical community saw antibiotics as "the magic bullet" for curing infections many decades ago, I see nutritional agents, including dietary supplements and food planning based on individual needs, as "the magic bullets" for building health, preventing disease, and slowing down the aging process in the future. The most effective intervention to prevent chronic degenerative diseases will occur through matching a diet and exercise regimen to suit an individual's genetic make-up and susceptibility to each disease. Nutritionists concerned with over-nutrition (instead of malnutrition) for their clients should focus first and foremost on making dietary recommendations based on genetic predisposition.

It is time that a new medical model of lifestyle management becomes the most prominent component of healthcare in the twenty-first century. Researchers have the knowledge to focus on our genetic blueprint as the gold standard for optimizing our lifestyle. Eating real foods based on DNA compatibility could remove our risk for all degenerative diseases. That's what I call a "magic bullet"!

APPENDIX A

The "Feel Like a 10" Food Plan

The World Health Organization defines optimum health as *physical, mental, emotional and social well-being.* What we put into our bodies for fuel has everything to do with how we look, think, act, and feel. If a car can't run on the wrong fuel, how can we (the most perfect machines ever made) expect to operate efficiently?

Your **Personal Food Plan** incorporates healthy, minimally processed food choices in optimum portion sizes for four categories of food (protein, carbohydrates, fat, and free choices). Your ideal serving size recommendations should be discussed with your personal nutrition consultant and should be based on your height, weight, age, sex, body frame, and activity level. If you don't have advice from a personal nutrition consultant, the following table (see page 128) can give you an estimate of your optimum intake of protein, carbohydrate, and fat.

Blood type has also been incorporated into your Food Plan as follows:

Food Plan One is most compatible for Blood Type "O."

Food Plan Two is most compatible for Blood Type "A."

Food Plan Three is most compatible for Blood Type "B."

Food Plan Four is most compatible for Blood Type "AB."

The **Best Choices** may be consumed anytime. The **Worst Choices** should be eaten only occasionally, ideally no more than one from each sub-category (i.e. fish, meats/meat substitutes, grains, fruits, etc.) every four days. Any food that you know you are allergic to or don't digest well should be avoided completely. Choose a wide variety of foods to ensure absorption of a wide variety of nutrients and to prevent food intolerance.

Table of Daily Serving Portions for Adults

Portion A		**Portion E**	
Sex:	Male or Female	Sex:	Male or Female
Blood Type:	A, AB	Blood Type:	Any
Height:	5'7" or less	Height:	5'8" or more
Weight:	Overweight	Weight:	Overweight
Protein:	4-5	Protein:	5-6
Carbohydrates:	5-6	Carbohydrates:	4-5
Fat:	1-1½	Fat:	2
Portion B		**Portion F**	
Sex:	Male or Female	Sex:	Male or Female
Blood Type:	O,B	Blood type:	Any
Height:	5'7" or less	Height:	5'8" or more
Weight:	Overweight	Weight:	Normal or underweight
Protein:	5-6	Protein:	5-6
Carbohydrates:	4-5	Carbohydrates:	6-7
Fat:	1½	Fat:	2-2½
Portion C		**Portion G**	
Sex:	Female	Sex:	Male or Female
Blood Type:	Any	Blood Type:	Any
Height:	5'7" or less	Height:	5'8" or more
Weight:	Normal or underweight	Weight:	Underweight
Protein:	4-5	Protein:	6
Carbohydrates:	5-6	Carbohydrates:	7-8
Fat:	2	Fat:	2½-3
Portion D			
Sex:	Male		
Blood Type:	Any		
Height:	5'7" or less		
Weight:	Normal or underweight		
Protein:	4-5		
Carbohydrates:	6-7		
Fat:	2-2½		

Please note: Large-boned, muscular, and athletic individuals may need to **increase** their portions of protein, carbohydrate, and fat. People over the age of fifty or with a sedentary lifestyle may need to **decrease** their portions of protein, carbohydrate, and fat.

Food Plan One

Protein Choices

"Best Choices" (in suggested portions) may be consumed daily. "Worst Choices" should be consumed on a limited basis (preferably no more than one from each sub-category every 4 days or as otherwise directed by your healthcare professional).

Meat/Meat Substitutes: Fish/Seafood (from non-toxic waters)

Seafood Serving Sizes: 1 serving = 3 oz.

Best Choices

Abalone	Herring (fresh pick-	Pike	Sole
Albacore (tuna)	led or water)	Red Snapper	Sturgeon
Anchovy	Lox (nitrate-free)	Sailfish	Swordfish
Barracuda	Mackerel	Salmon	Tilapia
Beluga (caviar)	Mahimahi	Sardine	Trout
Catfish (farm-raised)	Monkfish	Sea Bass	Tuna
Cod (scrod)	Octopus	Shark	Yellowtail
Conch	Orange Roughy	Smelt	Whitefish (farm-
Grouper	Perch	Snail	raised)

Worst Choices

Bass	Eel	Halibut	Shad
Bluefish	Flounder	Lobster	Shrimp
Clam	Frog	Mussels	Squid (calamari)
Crab	Haddock	Oyster	Tilefish
Crayfish	Hake	Scallop	Turtle

Meat/Meat Substitutes: Meat/Poultry (all free range, Kosher, or organic)

Egg Serving Size:	*1 serving = 1 yolk plus 3 or 4 egg whites*
Poultry Serving Size:	*1 serving = 2 oz.*
Meat Serving Size:	*1 serving = 2 oz.*

Best Choices - Lean varieties

Beef	Game Meats	Quail
Buffalo	Lamb	Rabbit
Chicken	Mutton	Turkey
Chicken Eggs	Ostrich	Turkey Eggs
Cornish Hen	Partridge	Veal
Duck	Pheasant	Venison
Duck Eggs	Pork	

Worst Choices

Bacon (nitrate-free)	Goose	Liver
Canadian Bacon (nitrate-free)	Goose Eggs	Sausage (nitrate free)
	Ham (nitrate-free)	

Meat/Meat Substitutes: Non-animal proteins

Count each bean serving as 1 serving of carbohydrates for weight loss.

Please note: Beans are a common food sensitivity problem for Blood Type Os when consumed on a daily basis.

Best Choices

Beans (azuki, black, broad, cannellini, fava, pinto, white) - 1 cup cooked
Peas (black-eyed, split) -1 cup cooked
Protein Concentrate (rice, soy, egg) - 1 T.

Soyburger (high protein) - 1 patty
Tempeh- ½ cup cooked
Tofu, firm drained - 1 cup

Worst Choices

Beans (garbanzo, kidney, lentil, lima, navy, red, tamarind) - 1 cup cooked

Meat/Meat Substitutes: Dairy/Dairy Substitutes

(Organic or Imported Choices Only)
1 dairy servings recommended daily = ½ protein serving

Best Choices

Farmer's cheese - 2 oz.
Feta Cheese – 1½ oz.
Goat Cheese – 1½ oz.

Mozzarella Cheese, lowfat - 1 oz.
Soycheese, lowfat – 1½ oz.
Soymilk - 2 eight oz. glasses

Worst Choices

American Cheese (no artificial color) 1½ oz.
Blue Cheese – 1½ oz.
Buttermilk – 8 oz.
Camembert Cheese – 1½ oz.
Cheddar Cheese – 1½ oz.
Colby Cheese – 1½ oz
Cottage Cheese, lowfat - ½ cup
Edam Cheese – 1½ oz.
Goat's Milk - eight oz.
Gouda Cheese – 1½ oz.

Gruyere Cheese – 1½ oz.
Havarti Cheese – 1½ oz.
Jarlsberg Cheese – 1½ oz.
Kefir - 8 oz.
Milk (1% skim) - eight oz.
Monterey Jack Cheese - 2 oz.
Munster Cheese - 2 oz.
Provolone Cheese – 1½ oz.
Ricotta Cheese, lowfat - ½ cup.
Swiss Cheese - 2 oz.
Yogurt-lowfat, non fat 8 oz.

Carbohydrate Choices

"Best Choices" (in suggested portions) may be consumed daily. "Worst Choices" should be consumed on a limited basis (preferably no more than one from every sub-category every four days is suggested or as otherwise directed by your healthcare professional).

Grain/Grain Substitutes

Best Choices

Bread, sprouted grain
(Essene, Ezekiel, Manna) - 1 slice
Flour (quinoa, rice, soy) - ½ cup
Quinoa (grain, cereal, pasta) - ½ cup cooked

Pasta (Jerusalem artichoke, rice) - ¾ cup
Rice (converted, brown, hot cereal, pasta not enriched) - ½ cup cooked
Rice (bread, waffle, crackers) - 1 slice bread/waffle or 5 small crackers

Best Choices (continued)

Rice (cakes) - 2 large

Rice (dry cereal) - ¾ cup

Tapioca - ¾ cup cooked

Wild Rice - ½ cup cooked

Worst Choices

Alcohol (grain alcohol, beer) - 1.5 oz./
12 oz. beer

Amaranth - ½ cup cooked

Bagel/Bialy - ½ bagel or whole bialy

Barley - ½ cup cooked

Buckwheat (kasha, soba noodles) -
½ cup cooked

Bulgur - ½ cup cooked

Corn cereal, grits, pasta - ½ cup
cooked

Corn Chips (non-hydrogenated), dry
cereal - 1 cup

Corn taco, tortilla - 1 medium

Couscous - ½ cup. cooked

English Muffin - 1 half

Flour (barley, buckwheat, cornmeal, oat,
rye, whole wheat, white) - ½ cup

Hamburger/hot dog bun - 1 half

Kamut - ½ cup cooked

Matzoh - ½ square

Millet - ½ cup cooked

Oatmeal / Oat bran - ½ cup cooked

Popcorn (air-popped) - 2 cups lowfat

Pretzels - 1 cup lowfat

Pumpernickel bread - 1 slice

Rye(bread, crackers) -1 slice or 5 small
crackers

Semolina (durum wheat) - ½ cup
cooked

Spelt cereal - ½ cup cooked

Spelt bread - 1 slice

Tabouli - ½ cup cooked

Wheat (pasta, cereal) - ½ c. cooked,
¾ c. cereal

Wheat Bread (whole wheat, white,
tortilla) - 1 slice

Fruit / Fruit Juices (fresh squeezed)

Best Choices

Alcohol - wine - 5 oz. maximum
(preferably sulfite-free)

Apricot - ¼ cup dried, 2 small
raw/cooked

Apple - 1 medium

Banana - 1 medium

Berries (blackberry, blueberry, boysenberry, cranberry, elderberry, gooseberry, logon berry, raspberry,
strawberry) - ¾ cup

Cherries - ¾ cup

Currants - ¼ cup dried

Dates/Figs - ¼ cup dried

Grapefruit - ½ medium

Grapes - 1 cup

Guava - ½ medium

Juice (fresh squeezed from "Best"
choices) - ¾ cup

Kiwi - 1 medium

Kumquat - 1 medium

Lemon/Lime - unlimited

Mango - ½ slice

Melon (casaba, crenshaw, watermelon)
- 1 small slice

Nectarine - 1 medium

Papaya - ½ medium

Peach - 1 medium

Pear (Bartlett, Bosc, Asian) - 1 medium

Persimmon - 1 medium

Pineapple - ¾ cup

Plum - 2 small

Pomegranate - ½ medium

Prunes - ¼ cup dried

Raisins - ¼ cup dried

Starfruit - 1 medium

Worst Choices

Alcohol (cordial - 5 oz. maximum)
Coconut - ½ medium
Juice (from concentrate) - ¾ cup
Melon (Cantaloupe, Honeydew) - 1
   small slice

Orange - 1 medium
Plaintain - 1 medium
Sorbet (ice) no added sugar - ½ cup
Tangelo - 1 medium
Tangerine - 2 small

High Starch Vegetables

Best Choices

Artichoke - 1 whole
Asparagus - 1 cup
Bamboo shoots - ¾ cup cooked
Beans (green, snap) - ¾ cup cooked;
   dry (see "non-animal" proteins)
Beets - ½ cup
Broccoli - 1 cup cooked
Brussels Sprouts - 1 cup cooked
Carrot - ½ cup cooked, 1 large raw,
   8 baby
Cucumber - ¾ cup
Jicama - ¾ cup

Kohlrabi - ¾ cup
Palm, hearts of - ¾ cup
Parsnip - 1 large raw, cooked
Peas, green - ¾ cups cooked
Potato, sweet - 1 medium
Sauerkraut (naturally fermented) - ¾ cup
Squash (acorn, spaghetti) - ¾ cup
Tofu - 1 cup
Turnip - ¾ cup
Water Chestnuts - ¾ cup
Yam - 1 medium
Zucchini - ¾ cup

Worst Choices

Cabbage - 1 cup cooked
Cauliflower - 1 cup cooked
Corn, kernel - ½ cup cooked, 1 large
   corn-on-the-cob
Eggplant - ¾ cups cooked

Pickles (naturally fermented)- ⅓ cup
Potato - white (English)- 1 medium
Potato - french fries, baked - 1 cup
Potato - chips, non-hydrogenated - 1 cup

Simple Sugars
(one maximum serving daily)

Best Choices

Date sugar/syrup - 1 T.
Fig syrup - 1 T.
Fruit Spread - 1 T.
Honey, raw - 1 T.
Maple Syrup, pure - 1 T.
Molasses (black strap, unsulphured) - 1 T.

Rice Syrup - 1 T.
Sorbet (ice) no added sugar - ½ cup
Sucanat – 1 T
Sugar, raw, liquid cane - 1 T.
Stevia - unlimited

Worst Choices

Barley malt - 1 T.
Corn sugar, syrup - 1 T.
Honey, commercial, cooked - 1 T.
Jam/Jelly - 1 T.
Juice Drinks (w/ added sugar) - ¾ cup
Sherbet - ½ cup

Soft Drink - 12 oz. maximum natural,
   no phosphoric acid
Sports Drink - 12 oz. max., no artificial
   colors
Yogurt, frozen - ½ cup

Fat Choices

"Best Choices" (in suggested portions) may be consumed daily. "Worst Choices" should be consumed on a limited basis (no more than one from every sub-category every four days is suggested or as otherwise directed by your healthcare professional).

Best Choices

Almond (nut/butter/oil) - ¼ cup raw/dry roasted 2 T. butter - 1 T. oil,

Butter, organic - 2 T. whipped / 1 T. stick

Canola (oil / margarine, non hydrogenated) 1 T.

Chocolate - 2 oz. pure (milk-free)

Chestnuts - ¼ cup raw/dry roasted

Filbert nuts - ¼ cup raw/dry roasted

Flax (seeds/oil) - ¼ cup seed - 1 T. oil

Ghee - 1 T. (Clarified butter)

Hickory nuts - ¼ cup raw / dry roasted

Hummus (full-fat) - ¼ cup

Macadamia nuts - ¼ cup raw / dry roasted

Olive (fruit/oil) - 6 large fruit - 1 T. oil

Pecans - ¼ cup raw/dry roasted

Pine nuts (pignola) - ¼ cup raw/dry roasted

Pumpkin seeds - ¼ cup raw/dry roasted

Rice bran oil - 1 T.

Sesame (seeds/butter(tahini)/oil) - ¼ cup raw/dry roasted - 2 T. butter, 1 T. oil

Soy (oil, margarine, non-hydrogenated) - 1 T., soynuts - ½ cup

Sunflower (seeds/butter/oil) - ¼ cup raw/dry roasted - 2 T. butter, 1 T. oil

Walnuts - ¼ cup raw/dry roasted

Worst Choices

Avocado (fruit/oil) - ¼ medium (large or small) - 1 T. oil

Brazil nuts - ¼ cup raw/ dry roasted

Cashew (nut/butter/oil) - ¼ cup raw/dry roasted - 2 T. butter, 1 T. oil

Corn (oil, margarine) 1 T.

Cottonseed oil - 1 T.

Cream Cheese, organic - 2 T.

Guacamole - ¼ cup

Ice Cream - ½ cup

Litchi nuts - ¼ cup raw/dry roasted

Peanut (nut/butter/oil) - ¼ cup raw/dry roasted - 2 T. butter, 1T. oil

Pistachio (nut/oil) - ¼ cup raw/dry roasted - 1 T. oil

Safflower (oil/margarine) - 1 T.

Free Choices

Portions are unlimited unless otherwise stated.

Low Starch Vegetables

Best Choices

Arugula

Beet Leaves

Bok Choy

Celery

Chicory

Endive

Escarole

Fennel

Greens (collard, dandelion, mustard)

Kale

Kelp

Leek

Lettuce

Okra

Onion family (green, red, white, yellow; garlic, leek, chives, scallion, shallot)

Peppers (green, jalapeno, red, yellow)

Radicchio

Radish

Rutabaga

Seaweed

Spinach

Sprouts

Tomato

Vegetable juice, low sodium - 8 oz. maximum

Worst Choices
Mushrooms
Rhubarb

Spices / Condiments (fresh, dry, liquid)

Best Choices

Almond extract
Allspice
Anise
Arrowroot
Basil
Bayleaf
Cardamom
Carob
Celery seed
Cheryil
Chives
Cilantro
Cloves
Cocoa Powder
Coriander
Cumin
Curry

Dill
Dulse
Garlic
Gelatin (plain)
Ginger
Horseradish
Lemon Juice
Marjoram
Mint
Miso
Mustard, dry
Onion
Oregano
Paprika
Parsley
Pepper (cayenne, red)
Peppermint

Rosemary
Saffron
Sage
Salt, sea - 1 tsp. maximum
Savory
Spearmint
Stevia
Tamari - 1 tsp. maximum
Tarragon
Tartar, cream of
Thyme
Turmeric
Worcestershire - 1 tsp. max

Worst Choices

Barbecue sauce - 1 T. maximum
Capers
Catsup - 1 T. maximum
Cinnamon
Cornstarch
Nutmeg

Parmesan Cheese - 1 T. maximum
Pepper (white, black)
Pimento
Poppyseeds
Relish

Sodium chloride (table salt) - 1 tsp. maximum
Soy Sauce - 1 tsp. maximum
Vanilla
Vinegar - 1 tsp. maximum
Wintergreen

Drinks/Miscellaneous

Best Choices
Coffee, decaf, regular - 2 cups max.
Lemon water
Seltzer water
Soda, club
Tea, herbal (ginger, ginseng, peppermint, raspberry, licorice chamomile, peppermint, rose hips, sarsaparilla, spearmint) - 2 cups max.
Vegetable juice, low sodium - 8 oz. maximum
Water, sparkling/plain (filtered, distilled, or spring) - 4–8 cups

Worst Choices
Tap water (chlorinated)
Tea, black-decaf/regular - 2 cups max
Tea, herbal (strawberry leaf, clover, rhubarb) - 2 cups maximum

Medicinal Herbs (capsules, tincures, teas)
Best used under direction of a licensed health care professional.

Best Choices

Catnip	Fenugreek	Rosehips
Cayenne	Ginseng	Saw Palmetto
Chamomile	Horehound	Slippery Elm
Dandelion	Licorice	White Willow Bark
Dong Quai	Milk thistle (silymarin)	Valerian root

Worst Choices

Aloe	Gentian	Shepherd's Purse
Burdock	Goldenseal	Strawberry Leaf
Clover	Saint John's Wort	Yellow dock
Echinacea	Senna	

Food Plan Two

Protein Choices

"Best choices" (in suggested portions) may be consumed daily. "Worst choices" should be consumed on a limited basis (no more than one from every sub-category every 4 days is suggested or as otherwise directed by your healthcare professional).

Meat/Meat Substitutes: Fish/Seafood (from non-toxic waters)
1 serving = 3 oz.

Best Choices

Abalone	Mahimahi	Sardine	Tilapia
Albacore (tuna)	Monkfish	Sea Bass	Trout
Cod (scrod)	Orange Roughy	Shark	Whitefish (farm-
Grouper	Perch	Smelt	raised)
Lox (smoked	Pike	Snail	Yellowtail
salmon;	Red Snapper	Sole	
nitrate-free)	Sailfish	Sturgeon	
Mackerel	Salmon	Swordfish	

Worst Choices

Anchovy	Eel	Octopus
Barracuda	Flounder	Oyster
Bass	Frog	Scallop
Beluga (caviar)	Haddock	Shad
Bluefish	Hake	Shrimp
Catfish	Halibut	Squid (calamari)
Clam	Herring - fresh, pickled or	Tilefish
Conch	fresh water only	Turtle
Crab	Lobster	
Crayfish (farm-raised)	Mussels	

Meat/Meat Substitutes: Meat/Poultry (free range, Kosher, or organic)

Egg Serving Size: 1 serving = 1 yolk plus 3 egg whites or 4 whites
Poultry Serving Size: 1 serving = 2 oz.
Meat Serving Size: 1 serving = 2 oz.

Best Choices - lean varieties

Chicken eggs	Cornish hen	Turkey eggs
Chicken	Turkey	

Worst Choices

Bacon (nitrate-free)	Goose	Pork
Beef	Goose Eggs	Pork
Buffalo	Ham (nitrate-free)	Quail
Canadian bacon	Lamb	Rabbit
(nitrate-free)	Mutton	Sausage (nitrate-free)
Duck	Ostrich	Veal
Duck eggs	Partridge	Venison
Game meats	Pheasant	

Meat/Meat Substitutes: Non-animal proteins

Count as 1 serving of carbohydrate for weight loss (if not vegetarian).

Best Choices

Beans (azuki, black, broad, cannellini fava, lentils, pinto, white) - 1 cup cooked	Soyburger (high protein) - 1 patty
	Soynuts - ½ cup
	Tempeh - ½ cup cooked
Peas (black-eyed, split) - 1 cup cooked	Tofu, firm drained - 1 cup
Protein Concentrate (rice, soy, egg) - 1 scoop	

Worst Choices

Beans (garbanzo, kidney, lima, navy, red, tamarind) - 1 cup cooked

Meat/Meat Substitutes: Dairy/Dairy Substitutes

Organic or Imported Choices Only.
2 dairy servings (maximum daily) - 1 protein serving

Best Choices

Cottage cheese (lowfat) - ½ cup	Mozzarella cheese, lowfat - 1 oz.
Farmer's cheese - 2 oz.	Ricotta cheese, lowfat - ½ cup
Feta cheese - 1½ oz.	Soycheese, lowfat - 1½ oz.
Goat's cheese - 1½oz.	Soymilk - 8 oz. glass
Goat's milk - 8 oz.	Yogurt, lowfat or no fat - 8 oz.
Kefir - 8 oz. glass	

Worst Choices

American cheese (free of artificial color) - 1½ oz	Camembert cheese - 1½ oz.
	Cheddar cheese - 1½ oz.
Blue cheese - 1½ oz.	Colby cheese - 1½ oz.
Brie - 1½ oz.	Edam cheese - 1½ oz.
Buttermilk - 8 oz. glass	Gouda cheese - 1½ oz.

Worst Choices (continued)
Gruyere cheese - 1½ oz.
Havarti - 1½ oz.
Jarlsberg cheese - 1½ oz.
Milk (1%, skim) - 8 oz. glass

Monterey Jack cheese - 1½ oz.
Munster cheese - 1½ oz.
Provolone cheese - 1½ oz.
Swiss cheese - 1½ oz.

Carbohydrate Choices
"Best choices" (in suggested portions) may be consumed daily. "Worst choices" should be consumed on a limited basis (no more than one from every sub-category every 4 days is suggested or as otherwise directed by your healthcare professional).

Grain/Grain Substitutes

Best Choices
Barley, pearled - ½ cup cooked
Bread, sprouted grain (Essene, Ezekiel, manna) - 1 slice
Buckwheat (kasha, soba noodles) - ½ cup cooked
Corn cereal, grits, pasta - ½ cup cooked, 3/4 cup cereal
Corn taco, tortilla - 1 medium
Corn chips (non-hydrogenated), dry cereal - 1 cup
Flour (barley, buckwheat, cornmeal, oat, quinoa, rye, rice, soy) - ½ cup
Kamut - ½ cup cooked
Millet - ½ cup cooked
Oatmeal/Oat bran - ½ cup cooked
Pasta (Jerusalem artichoke, rice, soba) - ¾ cup

Popcorn (air-popped) - 2 cups lowfat
Pumpernickel bread - 1 slice
Quinoa (grain, cereal, pasta) - ¾ cup cooked
Rice (converted, brown, hot cereal, pasta) - ½ cup cooked
Rice (cakes) - 2 large
Rice (bread, crackers and waffle) - 1 slice or 5 small crackers
Rice (dry cereal) - ¾ cup
Rye (bread, crackers) - 1slice or 5 small crackers
Semolina (durum wheat) - ½ cup cooked or - 1 slice semolina bread
Tapioca - ¾ cup cooked
Wild Rice - ½ cup cooked

Worst Choices
Alcohol (beer) - 12 oz. maximum
Alcohol (grain alcohol) - 1.5 oz. maximum.
Amaranth - ½ cup cooked
Bagel/bialy - ½ bagel or whole bialy
Bulgur - ½ cup cooked
Couscous - ½ cup cooked
English muffin - 1 half
Flour (whole wheat, white) - ½ cup
Hamburger/hot dog bun - 1 half
Matzoh - ½ square

Pretzels - 1 cup lowfat
Rice (white) - ½ cup cooked
Spelt cereal - ½ cup cooked
Spelt bread - 1 slice
Tabouli - ½ cup cooked
Triticale - ½ cup cooked
Wheat (pasta, cereal) - ½ cup cooked pasta - ¾ cup dry cereal
Wheat Bread (whole wheat, white, tortilla) - 1 slice

Fruit/Fruit Juices (fresh squeezed)

Best Choices

Alcohol (wine) - 5 oz. maximum.
  (preferably sulfite-free)
Apricot - ¼ cup dried, 2 small
  raw/cooked
Apple - 1 medium
Berries (blackberry, blueberry, boysen-
  berry, cranberry, elderberry, goose-
  berry, logon berry, raspberry,
  strawberry) - ¾ cup
Cherries - ¾ cup
Currants - ¼ cup dried
Dates/Figs - ¼ cup dried
Grapefruit - ½ medium
Grapes - 1 cup
Guava - ½ medium
Juice (fresh squeezed from "Best"
  choices) - ¾ cup

Kiwi - 1 medium
Kumquat - 1 medium
Lemon/Lime - unlimited
Mango - ½ slice
Melon (casaba, crenshaw, watermelon)
  - 1 small slice
Nectarine - 1 medium
Peach - 1 medium
Pear (Bartlett, Bosc, Asian) - 1 medium
Persimmon - 1 medium
Pineapple - ¾ cup
Plum - 2 small
Pomegranate - ½ medium
Prunes - ¼ cup dried
Raisins - ¼ cup dried
Starfruit - 1 medium

Worst Choices

Alcohol (cordial) - 5 oz. maximum)
Banana - 1 medium
Coconut - ½ medium
Juice (from concentrate) - ¾ cup
Mango - ½ slice
Melon (cantaloupe, honeydew)
  - 1 small slice

Orange - 1 medium
Papaya - ½ cup medium
Plaintain - 1 medium
Sorbet (ice), no added sugar) - ½ cup
Tangelo - 1 medium
Tangerine - 2 small

High Starch Vegetables

Best Choices

Artichoke - 1 whole
Bamboo shoots - 3/4 cup cooked
Beans (green, snap, soy) - 3/4 cup
  cooked
Beans, dry (see "non-animal" proteins)
Beets - ½ cup
Broccoli - 1 cup cooked
Brussels Sprouts - 1 cup cooked
Carrot - ½ cup cooked, 1 large raw,
  8 baby
Cauliflower - 1 cup cooked
Corn, kernal - ½ cup cooked, 1 large
  corn-on-the cob
Cucumber - ¾ cup

Jicama - ¾ cup
Kohlrabi - ¾ cup
Palm, hearts of - ¾ cup
Parsnip - 1 large raw, cooked
Peas, green - ¾ cups cooked
Potato, sweet - 1 medium
Pumpkin - ¾ cup
Sauerkraut (naturally fermented) - ¾ cup
Squash (acorn, spaghetti) - ¾ cup
Turnip - ¾ cup
Water Chestnut - ¾ cup
Yam - 1 medium
Zucchini - ¾ cup

Worst Choices

Asparagus - 1 cup
Cabbage - 1 cup cooked
Eggplant - ¾ cup cooked
Pickles (naturally fermented) - ⅓ cup

Potato- white (English) - 1 medium
Potato chips, non hydrogenated - 1 cup
Potato, french fries (baked) - 1 cup

Simple Sugars
one maximum serving daily

Best Choices

Date sugar/syrup - 1 T.
Fig syrup - 1 T.
Fruit Spread - 1 T
Honey, raw - 1 T.
Maple Syrup, pure - 1 T.
Molasses (black strap, unsulphured) - 1 T.

Rice Syrup - 1 T.
Sorbet (ice), no added sugar) - ½ cup
Sucanat - 1 T.
Sugar, raw, liquid cane - 1 T
Stevia - unlimited
Yogurt, frozen- ½ cup

Worst Choices

Barley malt - 1 T.
Corn sugar, syrup - 1 T.
Honey, commercial, cooked - 1 T.
Jam/Jelly - 1 T.
Juice Drinks (w/ added sugar) - ¾ cup
Sherbet (no artificial colors/flavors)
   - ½ cup

Soft Drink - 12 oz. maximum natural,
   no phosphoric acid
Sports Drink - 12 oz. max., no artificial
   colors
Sugar, beet, brown, cane - 1 T.

Fat Choices

"Best choices"(in suggested portions) may be consumed daily. "Worst choices" should be consumed on a limited basis (no more than one from every sub-category every 4 days is suggested or as otherwise directed by your healthcare professional).

Best Choices

Almond (nut/butter/oil) - 1/4 cup raw/dry roasted - 2 T. butter,1 T. oil
Avocado (fruit/oil) - 1/4 medium (large or small) - 1 T. oil
Canola (oil/margarine, non-hydrogenated) - 1 T.
Chestnuts - ¼ cup raw/dry roasted
Filbert nuts - ¼ cup raw/dry roasted
Flax (seeds/oil) - ¼ cup seeds, 1 T. oil
Ghee - 1 T. (clarified butter)
Guacamole - ¼ cup
Hickory nuts - ¼ cup raw / dry roasted
Hummus (full-fat) - ¼ cup
Litchi nuts - ¼ cup raw/dry roasted
Macadamia nuts - ¼ cup raw / dry roasted
Olive (fruit/oil) - 6 large fruit, 1 T. oil
Pecans - ¼ cup raw / dry roasted
Peanut (nut/butter/oil) - ¼ cup
   raw/dry roasted, 2 T., butter, 1 T. oil
Pine nuts (pignola) - ¼ cup raw/dry roasted

Pumpkin seeds - ¼ cup raw/dry roasted
Rice bran oil - 1 T.
Sesame (seeds/butter(tahini)/oil) - ¼ cup raw/dry roasted, 2 T. butter, 1 T. oil
Soy (oil, margarine, non-hydrogenated) - 1 T.
Sunflower (seeds/butter/oil) - ¼ cup raw/dry roasted, 2 T. butter, 1 T. oil
Walnuts - ¼ cup raw/dry roasted

Worst Choices
Butter, organic - 2 T. whipped/1 T. stick
Brazil nuts - ¼ cup raw/dry roasted
Cashew (nut/butter/oil) - ¼ cup raw/dry roasted, 2 T. butter, 1 T. oil
Chocolate - 2 ounces pure (milk-free)
Corn (oil/margarine) - 1 T.
Cottonseed oil - 1 T.
Cream cheese, organic - 2 T.
Ice Cream - ½ cup
Mayonnaise - 1 T. reduced fat
Pistachio (nut/oil) - ¼ cup raw/dry roasted, 1 T. oil
Safflower (oil/margarine) - 1 T.

Free Choices
Portions are unlimited unless otherwise stated.

Low Starch Vegetables

Best Choices

Arugula	Greens (collard,	Radicchio
Beet Leaves	dandelion, mustard)	Radish
Bok Choy	Kale	Rutabaga
Celery	Kelp	Seaweed
Chicory	Leek	Spinach
Cilantro	Lettuce	Sprouts
Endive	Okra	Swiss chard
Escarole	Onion family (green, red,	Watercress
Fennel	white, yellow; garlic,	
	leek, chives, scallion,	
	shallot)	

Worst Choices

Mushrooms	Rhubarb	Vegetable juice, (low
Peppers (green, jalapeno,	Tomato	sodium) - 8 oz. maximum
red, yellow)		

Spices/Condiments (fresh, dry, liquid)

Best Choices

Almond extract	Cardamom	Cinnamon
Allspice	Carob	Cloves
Anise	Celery seed	Cocoa Powder
Arrowroot	Chervil	Coriander
Basil	Chives	Cumin
Bayleaf	Cilantro	Curry

Best Choices (continued)

Dill	Nutmeg	Spearmint
Dulse	Onion	Stevia
Garlic	Oregano	Tamari - 1 T. maximum
Gelatin (plain)	Parmesean Cheese - 1 T.	Tarragon
Ginger	Parsley	Tartar, cream of
Horseradish	Peppermint	Thyme
Lemon Juice (fresh)	Rosemary	Turmeric
Marjoram	Saffron	Worcestershire - 1 T. max
Mint	Sage	Vanilla
Miso	Salt, sea - 1 tsp. maximum	
Mustard, dry	Savory	

Worst Choices

Barbecue Sauce - 1 T. maximum	Sodium chloride (table salt) - 1 tsp.
Capers	max
Catsup - 1 T. maximum	Soy sauce - 1 T. maximum
Cornstarch	Vinegar - 1 T. maximum
Pepper (cayenne, black, red, white)	Wintergreen
Pimento	

Drinks/Miscellaneous

Best Choices

Coffee, decaf/regular - 2 cups max
Lemon water
Tea, herbal (ginger, ginseng, peppermint, raspberry, licorice, strawberry leaf - 2 c.
Tea, black, green-decaf/regular - 2 cups maximum
Water, sparkling/plain (filtered, distilled, or spring) - 4–8 cups

Worst Choices

Seltzer water
Soda, club
Tap water (chlorinated)-
Tea, herbal (chamomile, clover, rose hips, rhubarb, sarsaparilla, spearmint) - 2 cups
    maximum
Tomato juice (low sodium) - 8 oz. max.

Medicinal Herbs (capsules, tinctures, tea)

Best Choices

Aloe	Fenugreek	Rosehips
Burdock	Gentian	Saw Palmetto
Dandelion	Horehound	Saint John's Wort
Dong Quai	Licorice	Senna
Echinachea	Milk thistle (silymarin)	Shepherd's Purse

Worst Choices

Catnip	Clover	White willow bark
Cayenne	Goldenseal	Yellow dock
Chamomile	Slippery elm	

Food Plan Three

Protein Choices

"Best choices" (in suggested portions) may be consumed daily. "Worst choices" should be consumed on a limited basis (no more than one from every sub-category every 4 days is suggested or as otherwise directed by your healthcare professional).

Meat/Meat Substitutes: Fish/Seafood (from non-toxic waters)

1 serving = 3 oz.

Best Choices

Abalone	Lox (smoked	Sailfish	Squid (calamari)
Albacore (tuna)	salmon);	Salmon	Sturgeon
Cod (scrod)	nitrate-free only	Sardine	Swordfish
Catfish	Mackerel	Scallop	Tilapia
Flounder	Mahimahi	Sea Bass	Tilefish
Haddock	Monkfish	Shad	Trout
Halibut	Orange Roughy	Shark	Tuna
Herring (fresh	Perch	Smelt	Whitefish (farm-
water only)	Pike	Sole	raised)
	Red snapper		

Worst Choices

Anchovy	Conch	Herring (fresh,	Shrimp
Barracuda	Crab	pickled)	Snail
Bass	Crayfish	Lobster	Turtle
Beluga (caviar)	Eel	Mussels	Yellowtail
Bluefish	Frog	Octopus	
Clam		Oyster	

Meat/Meat Substitutes: Meat/Poultry (free range, Kosher, or organic)

Egg Serving Size:	1 serving = 1 yolk plus 3 egg whites or 4 whites
Poultry Serving Size:	1 serving = 2 oz.
Meat Serving Size:	1 serving = 2 oz.

Best Choices - Lean Varieties

Beef	Game meats	Ostrich	Turkey
Buffalo	Goose eggs	Pheasant	Veal
Chicken eggs	Lamb	Pork	Venison
Duck eggs	Mutton	Rabbit	

Worst Choices

Bacon (nitrate-free)	Cornish hen	Liver (1 time per month)
Canadian bacon (nitrate-	Duck	Quail
free)	Goose	Sausage (nitrate-free)
Chicken	Ham (nitrate-free)	

Meat/Meat Substitutes: Non-animal proteins

Count as 1 serving of carbohydrate for weight loss (if not vegetarian)

Best Choices

Beans (broad, cannellini, fava, kidney, lima, navy, white) - 1 cup cooked
Protein Concentrate (rice, soy, egg) - 1 T.
Soyburger (high protein) - 1 patty

Worst Choices

Beans (Azuki, black, garbanzo, pinto, lentil, tamarind) - 1 cup cooked
Peas (black-eyed, split) - 1 cup cooked
Tempeh - ½ cup cooked
Tofu, firm drained - 1 cup

Meat/Meat Substitutes: Dairy/Dairy Substitutes

Organic or Imported Choices Only.
2 dairy servings = 1 protein serving
(Preferably from NON-CORN FED animals as in most imported milk products)

Best Choices

Brie - 1½ oz.
Buttermilk - 8 oz. glass
Camembert cheese - 1½ oz.
Cheddar cheese - ½ oz.
Colby cheese - 1½ oz.
Cottage cheese (lowfat) - ½ cup
Edam cheese - 1½ oz.
Farmer's cheese - 2oz.
Feta cheese - 1½ oz.
Goat's cheese - 1½ oz.
Goat's milk - 1½ oz.
Gouda cheese - 1½ oz.
Gruyere cheese- 1½ oz.

Havarti - 1½ oz.
Jarlsberg cheese - 1½ oz.
Kefir - 8 oz. glass
Milk (1%, skim) - 8 oz. glass
Monterey Jack cheese - 1½ oz.
Munster cheese - 1½ oz.
Provolone cheese - 1½ oz.
Ricotta cheese, lowfat - ½ cup
Soycheese, lowfat - 1½ oz.
Soymilk - 8 oz. glass
Swiss cheese - 1½ oz.
Yogurt, lowfat or no fat - 8 oz.

Worst Choices

American cheese (free of artificial color) - 1½ oz.
Blue cheese - 1½ oz.
Mozzarella cheese, lowfat - 1½ oz.

Carbohydrate Choices

"Best choices" (in suggested portions) may be consumed daily. "Worst choices" should be consumed on a limited basis (no more than one from every sub-category every 4 days is suggested or as otherwise directed by your healthcare professional).

Grain/Grain Substitutes

Best Choices

Amaranth - ½ cup cooked
Bread, sprouted grain (Essene, Ezekiel)
  - 1 slice

Couscous - ½ cup, cooked
Flour (oat, quinoa, rice, soy) - ½ cup
Millet - ½ cup cooked

Best Choices (continued)

Oatmeal/ Oat bran - ½ cup cooked
Pumpernickel bread - 1 slice
Quinoa (grain, cereal, pasta) - ½ cup cooked
Rice (bread, crackers, waffle) - 1 slice/waffle or 5 small crackers
Rice (converted, brown, pasta, hot cereal) - ½ cup cooked

Rice cakes - 2 large cakes/bread, crackers - 1 slice or 5 small crackers
Rice cereal (dry) - ¾ cup
Semolina (durum wheat) - ½ cup cooked
Spelt bread - 1 slice
Spelt cereal - ½ cup cooked
Wild rice - ½ cup, cooked

Worst Choices

Alcohol (beer) - 12 oz., 1 maximum daily
Alcohol (grain) - 1.5 oz. maximum
Bagel/bialy - ½ bagel or whole bialy
Barley, pearled - ½ cup cooked
Buckwheat (kasha, soba noodles) - ½ c. cooked
Bulgur - ½ cup cooked
Corn taco, tortilla - 1 medium
Corn cereal, grits, pasta - ½ cup cooked, ¾ cup cold cereal
Corn chips (non-hydrogenated) - 1 cup
English muffin - 1 half
Flour (barley, buckwheat, cornmeal, rye, white) - ½ cup

Hamburger/hot dog bun - 1 half
Kamut - ½ cup cooked
Matzoh - ½ square
Pasta (Jerusalem artichoke, soba) - ¾ cup
Popcorn (air-popped) - 2 cups lowfat
Pretzels - 1 cup lowfat
Rye (bread, crackers) - 1 slice or 5 small crackers
Tabouli - ½ cup cooked
Tapioca - ¾ cup cooked
Wheat (pasta, cereal) - ½ cup cooked
Wheat bread (whole wheat, white, tortilla) - 1 slice

Fruit/ Fruit Juices (fresh squeezed)

Best Choices

Alcohol (wine) - 5 oz. max. (preferably sulfite-free)
Alcohol (cordial) - 2 oz. max.
Apricot - ¼ cup dried, 2 small raw/cooked
Apple - 1 medium
Banana - 1 medium
Berries (blackberry, blueberry, boysenberry cranberry, elderberry, gooseberry, logon berry, raspberry, strawberry) - ¾ cup
Cherries - ¾ cup
Currants - ¼ cup dried
Dates/Figs - ¼ cup dried
Grapefruit - ½ medium
Grapes - 1 cup
Guava - ½ medium
Juice (fresh squeezed from "Best" choices) - ¾ cup

Kiwi - 1 medium
Kumquat - 1 medium
Lemon/Lime - unlimited
Mango - ½ slice
Melon (casaba, crenshaw, cantaloupe, watermelon) - 1 small slice
Nectarine - 1 medium
Orange - 1 medium
Papaya - ½ medium
Peach - 1 medium
Pear (Bartlett, Bosc, Asian) - 1 medium
Pineapple - ¾ cup
Plaintain - 1 medium
Plum - 2 small
Prunes - ¼ cup dried
Raisins - ¼ cup dried
Tangelo - 1 medium
Tangerine - 2 small

Worst Choices

Coconut - ½ medium
Juice (from concentrate) - ¾ cup
Persimmon - 1 medium

Pomegranate - ½ medium
Star fruit - 1 medium
Sorbet (ice) no added sugar - ½ cup

High Starch Vegetables

Best Choices

Asparagus - 1 cup
Bamboo shoots - ¾ cup cooked
Beans (green, snap) - ¾ cup cooked; dry
(see "non-animal" proteins)
Beets - ½ cup
Broccoli - 1 cup cooked
Brussels Sprouts - 1 cup cooked
Carrot - ½ cup cooked, 1 large raw,
8 baby
Cauliflower - 1 cup cooked
Cucumber - ¾ cup
Eggplant - ¾ cup cooked
Jicama - ¾ cup

Kohlrabi - ¾ cup
Palm, hearts of - ¾ cup
Parsnip - 1 large raw, cooked
Peas, green - ¾ cups cooked
Potato, sweet - 1 medium
Potato, white (English) - 1 medium
Sauerkraut (naturally fermented) - ¾ cup
Squash (acorn, spaghetti) - ¾ cup
Turnip - ¾ cup
Water Chestnut - ¾ cup
Yam - 1 medium
Zucchini - ¾ cup

Worst Choices

Artichoke - 1 whole
Beans - see "non-animal proteins"
Corn, kernel - ½ cup, 1 large corn-on-
cob
Pickles (naturally fermented) - 1/3 cup

Potato chips, non-hydrogenated - 1 cup
Potato, french fries (baked) - 1 cup
Pumpkin - ¾ cup
Tempeh - 1 cup
Tofu - 1 cup

Simple Sugars

one maximum serving daily

Best Choices

Date sugar/syrup - 1 T.
Fig syrup - 1 T.
Fruit Spread - 1 T.
Honey, raw - 1 T.
Maple Syrup, pure - 1 T.
Molasses (black strap, unsulphured) - 1 T.

Rice Syrup - 1 T.
Sorbet (ice) no added sugar - ½ cup
Sucanat - 1 T.
Sugar, raw, liquid cane - 1 T.
Stevia - unlimited
Yogurt, frozen - ½ cup

Worst Choices

Barley malt - 1 T.
Corn sugar, syrup - 1 T.
Honey, commercial, cooked - 1 T.
Jam/Jelly - 1 T.
Juice Drinks (w/ added sugar) - ¾ cup
Sherbet - ½ cup

Soft Drink - 12 oz. maximum natural,
no phosphoric acid
Sports Drink - 12 oz. max., no artificial
colors
Sugar, beet, brown, cane - 1 T.

Fat Choices

"Best choices" (in suggested portions) may be consumed daily. "Worst choices" should be consumed on a limited basis (no more than one from every sub-category every 4 days is suggested or as otherwise directed by your healthcare professional).

Best Choices

Almond (nut/butter/oil) - ¼ cup raw/dry roasted, 2 T. butter, 1 T. oil
Brazil nuts - ¼ cup raw/dry roasted
Chestnuts - ¼ cup raw/dry roasted
Flax (seeds/oil) - ¼ cup seed, 1 T. oil
Ghee - 1 T. (clarified butter)
Hickory nuts - ¼ cup raw/dry roasted
Litchi nuts - ¼ cup raw/dry roasted
Macadamia nuts - ¼ cup raw/dry roasted

Olives (fruit, black or green) - 8 large fruit
Olive (oil) - 1 T.
Pecans - ¼ cup raw/dry roasted
Rice Bran oil - 1 T.
Soy (oil, margarine, non-hydrogenated) - 1 T., ½ cup soy nuts
Walnuts - ¼ cup raw/dry roasted

Worst Choices

Avocado (fruit/oil) - ¼ medium (large or small), 1 T. oil
Butter, organic - 2 T. whipped/ 1 T. stick
Canola (oil/margarine, non-hydrogenated) - 1 T.
Cashew (nut/butter/oil) - ¼ cup raw/dry roasted, 2 T. butter, 1 T. oil
Chocolate - 2 ounces pure
Corn (oil/margarine) - 1 T.
Cottonseed oil - 1 T.
Cream cheese, organic - 2 T.
Filbert nuts - ¼ cup raw/dry roasted
Guacamole - ¼ cup
Hummus (full fat) - ¼ cup
Ice cream - ½ cup

Margarine, any hydrogenated - 1 T.
Mayonnaise - 1 T. reduced fat
Peanut (nut/butter/oil) - ¼ cup raw/dry roasted, 2 T. butter, 1 T. oil
Pine nuts (pignola) - ¼ cup raw/dry roasted
Pistachio (nut/oil) - ¼ cup raw/dry roasted, 1 T. oil
Pumpkin seeds - ¼ cup raw/dry roasted
Safflower (oil/margarine) - 1 T.
Sesame (seeds/butter (tahini)/oil) - ¼ cup raw/dry roasted, 2 T. butter, 1 T. oil
Sunflower (seeds/butter/oil) - ¼ cup raw/dry roasted - 2 T. butter, 1 T. oil

Free Choices

Portions are unlimited unless otherwise stated.

Low Starch Vegetables

Best Choices

Arugula
Beet Leaves
Bok Choy
Celery
Chicory
Endive
Escarole
Fennel
Greens (collard, dandelion, mustard)
Kale

Kelp
Leek
Lettuce
    Sprouts (alfalfa,
Mushrooms
    broccoli, onion)
Okra
Onion family (green, red, white, yellow; garlic, leek, chives, scallion, shallot

Peppers (green, jalapeno, red, yellow)
Radicchio
Rutabaga
Seaweed
Spinach
Sprouts (alfalfa, broccoli, onion)
Swiss chard

Worst Choices

Radish	Tomato
Rhubarb	Tomato juice, low sodium - 8 oz. max.
Sprouts (radish, mung)	

Spices / Condiments (fresh, dry, liquid)

Best Choices

Almond extract	Cumin	Nutmeg	Sage
Anise	Curry	Onion	Salt, sea - 1 tsp.
Arrowroot	Dill	Oregano	max.
Basil	Dulse		Savory
Bayleaf	Garlic	Paprika	Spearmint
Capers	Ginger	Parmesan Cheese-	Stevia
Cardamon	Horseradish	1 T. max.	Tamari, 1 tsp. max.
Carob	Lemon juice (fresh)	Parsley	Tarragon
Celery seed	Marjoram	Pepper (cayenne,	Tartar, cream of
Chervil	Mint	red)	Thyme
Chives	Miso	Peppermint	Tumeric
Cilantro	Mustard, dry	Pimento	Wintergreen
Cloves	Mustard, commer-	Rosemary	Vanilla
Coriander	cial - 1T. max.	Saffron	Vinegar - 1 T. max.

Worst Choices

Allspice	Gelatin (plain)
Barley Malt	Poppyseed
Barbecue Sauce - 1 T. max.	Sodium chloride (table salt) - 1 tsp.
Catsup - 1 T. max.	Soy Sauce - 1 tsp. max
Cinnamon	Worcestershire sauce - 1 tsp. max.
Cornstarch	

Drinks/Miscellaneous

Best Choices

Coffee, decaf/regular - 2 cups max
Lemon water
Tea, herbal (chamomile, ginger, ginseng, peppermint, raspberry, licorice, rose hips, sarsaparilla, spearmint) - 2 c.
Tea, black, green-decaf/regular - 2 cups maximum
Water, sparkling/plain (filtered, distilled, or spring) - 4–8 cups

Worst Choices

Seltzer water
Soda, club
Tap water (chlorinated)
Tea, herbal (clover, rhubarb, senna) - 2 cups maximum
Tomato choice - low sodium - 8 oz. max.

Medicinal Herbs (capsules, tinctures, tea)
Best used under direction of a licensed health professional.

Best Choices

Burdock	Echinacea	Milk thistle (sily-	White willow bark
Catnip	Ginseng	marin)	Valerian Root
Cayenne	Golden seal	Rose hip	Yellow dock
Chamomile	Hawthorn	Saint John's Wort	
Dandelion	Horehound	Saw Palmetto	
Dong Quai	Licorice	Slippery Elm	

Worst Choices

Aloe	Fenugreek	Senna
Clover	Gentian	Shepherd's Purse

Food Plan Four

Protein Choices

"Best choices" (in suggested portions) may be consumed daily. "Worst choices" should be consumed on a limited basis (no more than one from every sub-category every 4 days is suggested or otherwise directed by your healthcare professional).

Meat/Meat Substitutes: Fish/Seafood (from non-toxic waters)
1 serving = 3 oz.

Best Choices

Abalone	Orange Roughy	Shark
Albacore (tuna)	Perch	Smelt
Cod (scrod)	Pike	Squid (calamari)
Catfish	Red snapper	Sturgeon
Halibut	Sailfish	Swordfish
Lox (smoked salmon; nitrate- free)	Salmon	Tilapia
	Sardine	Tilefish
Mackerel	Scallop	Trout
Mahimahi	Sea Bass	Tuna
Monkfish	Shad	Whitefish (farm-raised)

Worst Choices

Anchovy	Crayfish	Octopus
Barracuda	Eel	Oyster
Bass	Flounder	Shrimp
Beluga (caviar)	Haddock	Snail
Bluefish	Herring (fresh, pickled, or fresh water only)	Sole
Clam		Turtle
Conch	Lobster	Yellowtail
Crab	Mussels	

Meat/Meat Substitutes:
Meat/Poultry (free range, Kosher, or organic)

Egg Serving Size: 1 serving = 1 yolk plus 3 egg whites or 4 whites
Poultry Serving Size: 1 serving = 2 oz.
Meat Serving Size: 1 serving = 2 oz.

Best Choices - Lean Varieties

Chicken eggs	Mutton	Turkey
Duck eggs	Ostrich	Turkey eggs
Goose eggs	Pheasant	
Lamb	Rabbit	

Worst Choices

Bacon (nitrate-free)	Cornish Hen	Partridge
Beef	Duck	Pork
Buffalo	Game meats	Quail
Canadian bacon (nitrate-free)	Goose	Sausage (nitrate-free)
	Ham (nitrate-free)	
Chicken	Liver - 1 time monthly max	

Meat/Meat Substitutes: Non-animal proteins

Count as 1 serving of carbohydrate for weight loss or if not vegetarian.
Maximum serving daily.

Best Choices

Beans (broad, cannellini, navy, white)
   - 1 cup cooked
Protein Concentrate (rice, soy, egg)
   - 1 scoop

Soyburger (high protein) - 1 patty
Soynuts - ½ cup

Worst Choices

Beans (Azuki, black, fava, garbanzo,
   pinto, lentil, kidney, lima, tamarind)
   - 1 cup cooked

Peas (black eyed, split) - 1 cup cooked
Tempeh - ½ cup cooked
Tofu, firm, drained - 1 cup

Meat/Meat Substitutes: Dairy/Dairy Substitutes

Organic or Imported Choices Only.
2 dairy servings (maximum daily) = 1 protein serving

Best Choices

Cheddar cheese - 1½ oz.	Gouda cheese - 1½ oz.	Mozzarella cheese, lowfat - 1½ oz.
Colby cheese - 1½ oz.	Gruyere cheese - 1½ oz.	
Cottage cheese (lowfat) - ½ cup	Havarti - 1½ oz.	Ricotta cheese, lowfat - 2 oz.
	Jarlsberg cheese - 1½ oz.	
Edam cheese - 1½ oz.	Kefir - 8 oz. glass	Soycheese, lowfat - 1½ oz.
Farmer's cheese - 2oz.	Monterey Jack cheese - 1½ oz.	Soymilk - 8 oz. glass
Feta cheese - 1½ oz.		Swiss cheese - 1½ oz.
Goat's cheese - 1½ oz.	Munster cheese - 1½ oz.	Yogurt, lowfat or no fat - 8 oz.
Goat's milk - 1½ oz.		

Worst Choices

American cheese (free of artificial color)
  - 1½ oz.
Blue cheese - 1½ oz.
Brie - 1½ oz.

Buttermilk - 8 oz. glass
Camembert cheese - 1½ oz.
Milk (1%, skim) - 8 oz. glass
Provolone cheese - 1½ oz.

Carbohydrate Choices

"Best choices" (in suggested portions) may be consumed daily. "Worst choices" should be consumed on a limited basis (no more than one from every sub-category every 4 days is suggested or otherwise directed by your healthcare professional).

Grain/Grain Substitutes

Best Choices

Amaranth - ½ cup cooked
Barley, pearled - ½ cup cooked
Bread (whole & durum wheat, pita, tortilla) - 1 slice
Bread, sprouted grain (Essene, Ezekiel) - 1 slice
Bulgar - ½ cup cooked
Couscous - ½ cup
Flour (barley, oat, quinoa, rice, soy, whole wheat, rye) - ½ cup cooked
Millet - ½ cup cooked
Oatmeal/Oat Bran - ½ cup cooked
Pumpernickel bread - 1 slice
Quinoa (grain, cereal, pasta) - ½ cup cooked

Rice (converted, brown, pasta, hot cereal) - ½ cup cooked
Rice cakes - 2 large cakes/bread, crackers - 1 slice or 5 small crackers
Rice (bread, crackers, waffle) - 1 slice/waffle or 5 small crackers
Rye (bread, crackers) - 1 slice or 5 small crackers
Semolina (durum wheat) - ½ cup cooked or 1 slice semolina bread
Spelt cereal - ½ cup cooked
Spelt bread - 1 slice
Wheat (pasta, cereal) - ½ cup
Wheat bread (whole wheat, white, tortilla) - 1 slice

Worst Choices

Alcohol (beer) - 12 oz., 1 maximum daily
Alcohol (grain) - 1.5 oz., 1 maximum daily
Bagel/Bialy - ½ bagel or whole bialy
Buckwheat (kasha, soba noodles) - ½ cup
Corn taco, tortilla - 1 medium/
Corn chips - 1 c.
Corn cereal, grits, pasta - ½ cup cooked
English muffin - 1 half
Flour (buckwheat, cornmeal, white) - ½ cup

Hamburger/hot dog bun - 1 half
Kamut - ½ cup cooked
Kasha - ½ cup cooked
Matzoh - ½ square
Pasta (Jerusalem artichoke, soba) - ¾ cup
Popcorn (air popped) - 2 cups lowfat
Pretzels - ½ cup lowfat
Tabouli - ½ cup cooked
Tapioca - ¾ cup cooked

Fruit/ Fruit Juices (fresh squeezed)

Best Choices

Alcohol (wine) - 5 oz. max. (preferably sulfite-free)
Apricot - ¼ cup dried, 2 small raw/cooked
Apple - 1 medium

Berries (blackberry, blueberry, boysenberry cranberry, elderberry, gooseberry, logon berry, raspberry, strawberry) - ¾ cup

Cherries - ¾ cup
Currants - ¼ cup dried
Dates/Figs - ¼ cup dried
Grapefruit - ½ medium
Grapes - 1 cup
Juice (fresh squeezed from "Best" choices) - ¾ cup
Kiwi - 1 medium
Kumquat - 1 medium
Lemon/Lime - unlimited
Melon (casaba, crenshaw, cantaloupe, watermelon) - 1 small slice

Nectarine - 1 medium
Papaya - ½ medium
Peach - 1 medium
Pear (Bartlett, Bosc, Asian) - 1 medium
Pineapple - ¾ cup
Plantain - 1 medium
Plum - 2 small
Prunes - ¼ cup dried
Raisins - ¼ cup dried
Tangelo - 1 medium
Tangerine - 2 small

Worst Choices

Alcohol (cordial) - 1.5 oz. max. daily
Banana - 1 medium
Coconut - ½ medium
Guava - ½ medium
Juice (from concentrate) - ¾ cup
Mango - ½ slice

Orange - 1 medium
Pear (prickly) - 1 medium
Persimmon - 1 medium
Pomegranate - ½ medium
Sorbet (ice), no added sugar - ½ cup
Star fruit - 1 medium

High Starch Vegetables

Best Choices

Asparagus - 1 cup
Bamboo shoots - ¾ cup cooked
Beans (green, snap) - ¾ cup cooked
Beets - ½ cup
Broccoli - 1 cup cooked
Brussels Sprouts - 1 cup cooked
Cabbage - 1 cup cooked
Carrot - ½ cup cooked, 1 large raw, 8 baby
Cucumber - ¾ cup
Eggplant - ¾ cup cooked
Jicama - ¾ cup
Kohlrabi - ¾ cup

Palm, hearts of - ¾ cup
Parsnip - 1 large raw, cooked
Peas, green - ¾ cups cooked
Potato, sweet - 1 medium
Potato, white (English) - 1 medium
Pumpkin - ¾ cup
Sauerkraut (naturally fermented) - ¾ cup
Squash (acorn, spaghetti) - ¾ cup
Turnip - ¾ cup
Water Chestnut - ¾ cup
Yam - 1 medium
Zucchini - ¾ cup

Worst Choices

Artichoke - 1 whole
Beans (dry) - see "non animal proteins"
Corn, kernel - ½ c. cooked, 1 lg. corn-on-cob

Pickles (naturally fermented) - ⅓ cup
Potato chips, non hydrogenated - 1 cup
Potato, french fries (baked) - 1 cup

Simple Sugars
one maximum serving daily

Best Choices

Date sugar/syrup - 1 T.
Fig syrup - 1 T.
Fruit Spread - 1 T.
Honey, raw - 1 T.
Maple Syrup, pure - 1 T.
Molasses (black strap, unsulphured) - 1 T.

Rice Syrup - 1 T.
Sorbet (ice), no added sugar - ½ cup
Sucanat - 1 T.
Sugar, raw, liquid cane - 1 T.
Stevia - unlimited
Yogurt, frozen - ½ cup

Worst Choices

Barley malt - 1 T.
Corn sugar, syrup - 1 T.
Honey, commercial, cooked - 1 T.
Jam/Jelly - 1 T.
Juice Drinks (w/ added sugar) - ¾ cup
Sherbet - ½ cup

Soft Drink - 12 oz. maximum natural,
    no phosphoric acid
Sports Drink - 12 oz. max., no artificial
    colors
Sugar, beet, brown, cane - 1 T.

Fat Choices

"Best choices" (in suggested portions) may be consumed daily. "Worst choices" should be consumed on a limited basis (no more than one from every sub-category every 4 days is suggested or otherwise directed by your healthcare professional).

Best Choices

Almond (nut/butter/oil) - ¼ cup raw/dry
    roasted, 2 T. butter, 1 T. oil
Brazil nuts - ¼ cup raw/dry roasted
Cashew (nut/butter/oil) - ¼ cup raw/dry
    roasted, 2 T. butter, 1 T. oil
Chestnuts - ¼ cup raw/dry roasted
Flax (seeds/oil) - ¼ cup
Ghee - 1 T. (clarified butter)
Hickory nuts - ¼ cup raw/dry roasted
Litchi nuts - ¼ cup raw/dry roasted
Macadamia nuts - ¼ cup raw/dry roasted
Olives (fruit, black/oil) - 8 large fruit,
    1 T. oil

Peanut (nut/butter/oil) - ¼ cup raw/dry
    roasted, 2 T. butter, 1 T. oil
Pecans - ¼ cup raw / dry roasted
Pine nuts (pignola) - ¼ cup raw/dry
    roasted
Pistachio (nut/oil) - ¼ cup raw/dry
    roasted, - 1 T. oil
Pumpkin seeds - ¼ cup raw/dry roasted
Soy (oil, margarine, non-hydrogenated)
    - 1 T.
Walnuts - ¼ cup raw/dry roasted

Worst Choices

Avocado (fruit/oil) - ¼ medium (large
    or small), 1 T. oil
Chocolate - 2 ounces pure
Corn (oil/margarine) - 1 T.
Cottonseed oil - 1 T.
Cream cheese, organic - 2 T.
Filbert nuts - ¼ cup raw/dry roasted
Guacamole - ¼ cup
Hummus (full-fat) - ¾ cup
Ice cream - ½ cup

Margarine, any hydrogenated - 1 T.
Mayonnaise - 1 T. reduced fat
Olives (fruit, green with vinegar)
    - 8 large
Safflower (oil/margarine) - 1 T.
Sesame (seeds/butter (tahini)/oil) - 1/4 cup
    raw/dry roasted, 2 T. butter, 1 T. oil
Sunflower (seeds/butter/oil) - 1/4 cup raw/
    dry roasted, 2 T. butter, 1 T. oil

Free Choices

Portions are unlimited unless otherwise stated.

Low Starch Vegetables

Best Choices

Arugula
Beet Leaves
Bok Choy
Celery
Chicory
Endive
Escarole
Fennel
Greens (collard, dande-
    lion, mustard)
Kale

Kelp
Leek
Lettuce
Mushrooms (tree, oyster,
    portabello, Enoki)
Okra
Onion family (green, red,
    white, yellow, garlic,
    leek, chives, scallion,
    shallot)
Radicchio

Rutabaga
Seaweed
Spinach
Sprouts (alfalfa, broccoli,
    onion)
Swiss chard
Tomato

Worst Choices

Mushrooms (white, shitake)
Peppers (green, jalapeno, red, yellow)
Radish
Rhubarb

Sprouts (bean, mung, radish)
Tomato juice, low sodium-8 ounce
    maximum

Spices / Condiments (fresh, dry, liquid)

Best Choices

Almond extract
Arrowroot
Basil
Bayleaf
Cardamom
Carob
Celery seed
Chervil
Chives
Cilantro
Cloves
Coriander

Cumin
Curry
Dill
Dulse
Garlic
Ginger
Horseradish
Lemon juice (fresh)
Marjoram
Mint
Miso
Mustard, dry

Nutmeg
Onion
Oregano
Parmesan cheese
    - 1 T. max.
Parsley
Peppermint
Rosemary
Saffron
Sage
Salt, sea - 1 tsp.
    max.

Savory
Spearmint
Stevia
Tamari - 1 tsp. max.
Tarragon
Tartar, cream of
Thyme
Turmeric
Vanilla
Wintergreen

Worst Choices

Allspice
Anise
Barley malt
Barbecue sauce - 1 T.
    max.
Capers
Catsup - 1 T. max.

Cinnamon
Cornstarch
Gelatin (plain)
Paprika
Pepper (black/white, red,
    cayenne)
Pimento

Poppyseed
Sodium chloride (table
    salt) - 1 tsp. max.
Vinegar
Worcestershire sauce
    - 1 tsp. max.

Drinks / Miscellaneous

Best Choices
Coffee, decaf/regular - 2 cups max
Lemon water
Tea, black, green-decaf/regular - 2 cup
Tea, herbal (ginger, ginseng, peppermint, raspberry, licorice, rose hips, sarsaparilla)
  - 2 cups
Water, sparkling/plain (filtered, distilled, or spring) - 4–8 cups

Worst Choices
Seltzer water
Soda, club
Tap water (chlorinated) - 4–8 cups
Tea, herbal (chamomile, clover, rhubarb) - 2 cups. Max.
Tomato choice - low sodium, 8 oz. max.

Medicinal Herbs (capsules, tinctures, tea)
Best used under direction of a licensed health professional.

Best Choices

Burdock	Echinacea	Licorice	Saw Palmetto
Catnip	Ginseng	Milk Thistle	Slippery Elm
Cayenne	Golden Seal	(Silymarin)	White willow bark
Dandelion	Hawthorn	Rose hips	Valerian Root
Dong Quai	Horehound	Saint John's Wort	Yellow dock

Worst Choices

Aloe	Clover	Gentian	Shepherd's Purse
Chamomile	Fenugreek	Senna	

APPENDIX B
Natural Foods Shopping List

A Natural Foods Shopping List has been included to make it easy to find healthy brand names for your Best Choice foods. Most of these items can be found in large grocery stores, natural food markets, and/or health food stores. Due to the fact that food items are added and discontinued, please check our website at www.nutritionalconcepts.com where we will update this list every 6 months.

Breads/Muffins

Bob's Red Mill Creamy Rice Farina and other organic grain products
EnerG Tapioca bread (tapioca, safflower, sunflower oils, pear juice)
Heinneman's "Designer Crumpets"
Nakomi's Kamut Sourdough Bread
Baltic Bakery
Middle East Bakery
Nakomis (all varieties are great)

Natural Ovens of Manitowoc
Flax n' Honey
Brainy Bagels
English Muffin
24 Karrot Muffins
Pepperidge Farm Thick Dijon Rye and Pumpernickel
Rosen's Thin-cut Rye
Joseph's Pita

Pancakes/Waffles

Barbara Stitt's Pancake Mix (wheat-free also)
Van's Toaster waffles (one variety is wheat, gluten, egg, and yeast-free)

"No Yeast" Breads/Crackers

Blue Diamond Nut Thins (rice crackers with nutty flavors; wonderful!)
Ener-G Tapioca bread (gluten/yeast free)
Cedar's (thin white) Mountain Bread
Manischewitz Matzoh (garlic variety is great; now oat matzoh!)
Essene Rye or Wheat Bread (no yeast)
Ener-G-Rice Bread (yeast or no yeast)

French Meadows yeast-free, wheat-free Bread
Dumpftmeier Rye Bread (sourdough)
Boudin Sourdough (no yeast)
Ezekiel Bread (sprouted grains)
Manna Bread (sprouted grains, seeds, no yeast, no fat)

Grain Snacks
* Indicates high-in-fat but contains high quality oils with all natural ingredients

Cheese Puffs

Health Valley Cheddar Lites
Michael Season's Oat Bran Puffs

Barbara's Cheese Puffs (jalapeno and regular)

Corn Chips

Bearitos Corn Chips
*Barbara's Corn Chips/Barbara's Puffins
*El Jicente (taco style) Chips (many varieties include no salt)
Garden of Eden Little Soy Blues corn chips
Garden of Eden seven-grain tortilla chips

Michael Season's Oat Bran Tortillas (organically grown and high fiber)
*Tostito's brand 100% White Corn Restaurant Style Tortilla Chips
*Harry's Garden Beet-Garlic Corn Chips
Garden of Eatin' Corn Chips
Guiltless Gourmet (baked)

Potato/Rice/Veggie Chips

Michael Season's Shape-up Chips
Edward & Sons "Brown Rice Snaps" (for wheat allergies/gluten intolerance)
Ray's Taro Chips (great potato chip substitute for those who cannot tolerate potatoes)
Robert's American Gourmet Potato Flyers (Idaho potato, water, brown rice, canola oil, sea salt)
Guiltless Gourmet Chips
Saratoga Real Vegetable Chips (ingredients: Sweet Potato, Malanga Taro, Batata, Carrot, Yam, Yucca, Sunflower Oil)
Terra Chips (ingredients: Taro, Sweet Potato, Yuca, Batata, Parnsip, Taro colored with Beet Juice, Peanut Oil and/or Canola Oil, Sea Salt); delicious!
Potato Pops (ingredients: Potato Flour, Potato Starch, Water, Rice, Corn Bran, Safflower Oil, Salt, Natural Flavors); 1 gm. of fat
*Kettle (Potato)Chips

Popcorn

any brand popping corn (hulless corn can be popped in a paper lunchbag with no oil or a touch of canola and salt)
*Cape Cod White Cheddar Popcorn

Orville Redenbacher's lowfat varieties (some contain artificial color/flavor)
*Vic's Popping Corn
Bearitos Popping & Popped Corn

Pretzels

Barbara'a Whole Wheat Pretzels
East Shore Seasoned Pretzels
Oat Bran Pretzels

Snyder's Sourdough Pretzels
Nabisco (Fat Free) Mister Salty Pretzels
Newman's Own Organic Pretzels

Rice Cakes

Chico San (includes low and no sodium varieties)
Krispy Rice Cakes
Mini Rice Cakes

Quaker Oats Rice Cakes
American Grain "Rice Bites"
Hain (many varieties)
Lundberg Rice Cakes

Bakery and Delicatessen Items

Bagels (freshly made - not pre-packaged)
Bialys (freshly made - not pre-packaged)
Pasta (red sauce, touch of olive oil and vinegar; no cream sauces)
Cheese (light-colored cheeses; Lorraine Swiss and Alpine Lace are lowfat and low sodium)
Turkey Breast (lean, low sodium, no nitrite varieties)

***Sunset Gourmet, Bilmar, Jerome's, Applegate Farms Organic Turkey
Lean imported baked or boiled ham
Low-cal tuna or salmon salads
Fruit salad or vegetable salad (no sugar/ no mayo; oil/ vinegar/ lemon are great ingredients)
Applegate Farms hot dogs

Bakery and Delicatessen Items (continued)

The Pork Schop of Vermont uncured beef frankfurters and bratwurst (no artificial ingredients - great for kids)

Shelton's Turkey Sausage
Shelton's Turkey Jerky (regular and pepperoni flavor)

Pasta

DeBole's Jerusalem Artichoke Pasta (for those intolerant to whole wheat, high protein)
Edward & Son Oat Bran
Prince Superoni (high protein, wheat germ)
Papadini lentil pasta (gluten/wheat-free, delicious!)
Hodgson Mill Whole Wheat Pasta
semolina pasta (good brands include Al Dente, Antoine's, Duomo, Agnese, Fini, and Dececco)
Romance (refrigerator section, contains eggs)
Contadina (refrigerator section, contains eggs)

buckwheat noodles (Eden brand, Yamaimo Soba; great for people with wheat sensitivities)
China Bowl Rice Sticks (rice, water) and Cellophane Noodles (potato & green pea starch; great for grain and gluten intolerances)
rice noodles (check individual brands for additional ingredients.DeBole's is delicious)
Food for life 100% Rice Elbow Pasta
Pastariso Pasta (wheat/gluten free; made with organic rice)

Cooked Grains

Konriko Brand Wild Pecan rice
Arrowhead Mills "Quick-Cooking "brown rice
Uncle Ben's Converted Rice (the boil-in-bag variety is quick & easy)
Pritikin Rice and blends
tapioca (no wheat or gluten)
brown rice (any long or quick-cooking variety)
Kasha (made from buckwheat, good for wheat sensitive)

Texmati rice
Casbah "Nutted Pilaf"
Lundberg Rice Pilafs (300 mg. sodium)
Quinoa (good for grain sensitive, high protein)
Mother's Quick-Cooking barley (great for people with digestive problems and wheat sensitivities)
Lundberg Elegant Rice Pudding
Po River Valley Risotto

Cereals (Cooked and Uncooked)

**The best Cereal choices are high in fiber and contain less than 2 gms. of fat, less than 2 gms. of sucrose (and other refined sweeteners), and 300 mg. or less of sodium. ...check for added iron; if you' ve had any heart problems or cancer - you should avoid iron-enriched foods.

Erewhon Instant Oatmeal and Rice Twice cold cereal
Arrowhead Mills Organic Oatmeal (in pre-packaged serving bags)
oatmeal (old-fashioned or quick-cooking, not instant)
oat bran (good substitute for bread crumbs in recipes)
raw wheat germ
Nutri-Grain cereals

Shredded Wheat
Familia (green box)
Wheatena
Cream of Wheat
Cream of Rice
Quinoa hot cereal (good for wheat sensitive, high protein)
Kolln "Fruit n' Oat Bran Crunch" (no wheat, high fiber, very low sodium)
Puffed Kashi (seven grains)

Great Granola by "Natural Ovens of
  Manitowoc"
Puffed Wheat
Rice Chex
Puffed Rice
Rice Crispies
Grape Nuts
Perky's Nutty Rice Cereal
Cheerios
Erewhon Barley Plus
Breakfast Classics "Rice Crisps"

New Morning Cereals (most are wheat-
  free)
Fruit e' O's
Oat e' O's
Health Valley Cereals
Fiber 7
Fruit Lites
Oat Bran O's
Arrowhead Mills Puffed Millet & other
  varieties
Nature's Path Cereals

Crackers
Akmak (no yeast)
Ryvita toasted Sesame Rye (no wheat,
  very high fiber, no yeast)
Edward & Sons "Brown Rice Snaps"
  (brown rice, tamari, sesame seeds)
  - yeast free
Rye Krisp (unseasoned variety) - no yeast

Fiber (no yeast)
Kavli (no yeast)
Wasa (wheat, rye) - no yeast
Health Valley
Nature's Cupboard
rice cakes (most brands are O.K.) - no
  yeast

Taco Shells/Tortillas
Old El Paso Taco Shells
El Jinette Taco Chips (no salt variety)

tortillas (only those with corn, flour,
  water, lime, or a combination of these)

Flour and Baking Goods
Hodgson Mill flour
Arrowhead Mills flour
Elam flour
Ceresota Whole Wheat Flour
Stone Buhr flour
Barbara Stitt's Pancake Waffle Mix (milk
  and wheat-free)

Leavening Agents:
Arm & Hammer baking soda
Cellu Grain-Free or Featherweight
  Baking Powders (non-aluminum)

Thickeners

Tapioca	Potato Flour	Arrowroot Powder

Chocolate Substitutes
Carob powder (any brand)
Droste's or Hershey's unsweetened cocoa powder

Fruit Gelatin
Knox Gelatin (use with fruit juice for healthy, delicious "Jello")

Nuts and Seeds
(good for high-energy "kid" snacks; They contain no added fats or sodium if you get
  them in the baking section)

Jams and Sweeteners

Jams
Sorrell Ridge
Smucker's Simply Fruit or Fruit Spread
Polaner Fruit Spread

Spoon Fruit
Knudsen's Fruit Spread
Tree of Life

Corn Syrup/Pancake Syrup Substitutes
McDonald's Pure Maple Syrup
Shady Maple Farms Pure Maple Syrup
Grandma's Unsulphered Molasses
Brer Rabbit Unsulphered Molasses
Frozen apple juice concentrate (no
sugar added varieties)

Miss Figgy fig syrup
Honey (any brand if it is raw, unfiltered)
Rice Syrup (any brand)
Fig Pep fig syrup
Sucanat (organic granulated cane juice)
Date Sugar

White Sugar Substitutes
S & W Sugar-in-the-Raw (no chemical bleach)
Fructose (very light and powdery, low cal, may be tolerated by diabetics as ¼ fruit
exchange; DON'T USE IF CORN ALLERGIC)
Florida Crystals (unbleached) Cane Sugar

Sweets
Cookies, Muffins, Granola Bars
Natural Ovens of Manitowoc
muffins/cookies
BP Gourmet Cookies (very lowfat/low
sugar)
Callard & Bowser hard candy (2 pieces
daily max.)
Rendez-Vous or La Vosgienne Bon Bons
(delicious hard fruit and coffee can-
dies (no artificial colors/flavors)
R.W. Frookie cookies
Pamela's cookies (wheat-free/gluten free;
variety of flavors including simply
chocolate and pecan)
Glenny's Noah 'n Friends Animal
Cookies

Health Valley "Fat-Free" Cookies, "Fruit
Jumbos," "Oat Bran Graham Crackers,"
"Oat Bran Animal Cookies" (many
have low or no fat, most are fruit-juice
sweetened)
Barbara's cookies (fruit juice sweetened,
whole wheat)
Nature's Choice Granola Bars
Health Valley Granola Bars
Duchy's Originals (from England;
founded by the Prince of Whales;
use organic flour and no artificial
ingredients; many flavors; great dip-
ping cookies)

Fruit Desserts
Nature's Choice Real Fruit Bars (natural
answer to fruit roll-ups)
Dried fruits (choose sulfite-free)
Frookie Cool Fruits (frozen juice bars)
Canned fruit (canned-in-juice varieties)
Del Monte Pineapple Tidbits "Fruit
Cup" (Great for school lunches)
Koala Fruit Juice Bars (frozen; has corn)
Musselman's Natural Apple Sauce (snack
pack is great for school lunches)
Cherry Hill Organic Applesauce
- DELICIOUS
Santa Cruz organic applesauce (deli-
cious, snack packs are great for
school lunches)
Le Roux Creek Applesauce

Cascadian Farms Organic Sorbet
- DELICIOUS!
Nouvelle Sorbet (low cal, no sugar)
Frozen juice concentrates (can use as an
ingredient in desserts such as "Jello"
or can freeze for natural fruit pops)
Frozfruit Brand Frozen Fruit Bars
Fruitops (no added sugar)
Frookie "Cool Fruits" (no added sugar)
Nectar Freeze (70 calories, pure fruit)
Sweet Nothings (frozen fruit bars - GREAT!)
Seabrook frozen fruit (no added sugar)
Mama Tish Italian Ice (low calorie, sugar)
Mazzone's Soft Italian Sorbet (sugar)
Sensible Foods Fruit Snacks (dehydrated
fruits and veggies)

Candy and Gum

Panda Black Licorice (high iron, calcium, and B vitamins, made with real licorice root)

Finnfoods "Soft Licorice with Oat Bran" (high in B vitamins and calcium, made with real licorice root)

Natural (organic) Licorice Twists

Tropical Source drops (butterscotch, cherry, mint, papaya)

Tropical Source chocolates (many flavored bars and chocolate chips for baking)

Ford Extreme Xylitol gum

Trident Sugarless gum with baking soda

Speak Easy organic mints and gum (does contain cane juice, but wonderful!)

St. Claire's organic candies (cherry, cinnamon, ginger)

Sunspire chocolates (many kinds including peanuts, sundrops, raisins, etc.)

La Vosgienne Bonbons Fruits (many kinds including lemon, cherry, raspberry, cafe espresso, etc.)

Rendez Vous flavor candy (many kinds including sour lemon)

Frozen Confections (Dairy)

**The only safe dairy products are those that are certified organic or those that are imported because they are antibiotic/hormone free.

Gise Creme Glace (Sunset Yogurt Machine: imported from France; real fruit fructose, very low-cal)

Cascadian Farm frozen yogurt bars (98% fat free; only 80 calories per bar; organic; sweetened with Sucanat)

Homemade Yogurt: Whip your favorite organic nonfat yogurt with a ripe banana, freeze for 1–2 hours, delicious!

Jolle Yogurt

Stoneyfield Farms low fat ice-cream and frozen yogurt

Frozen Confections (Non-Dairy)

Rice Dream Non-dairy Dessert (high fat)

Rice Dream Chocolate or Carob drink boxes (freeze for 1–2 hours, tastes like a fudgesicle)

Oatscream frozen dessert

Nutty Rice Dream Bar (high in fat)

Imagine Foods "Dream Pudding"

Tofutti Light

Tofutti "Cuties" (delicious "ice cream" sandwiches)

Diana's Bananas

M&B Cool Snacks Banana Bites (bite size chocolate/nut covered bananas)

Doughnuts

Eggless Doughnut (no additives, no animal fat, no preservatives, no refined sugars, high in unsaturated fats)

Doughnuts (no dairy, wheat, eggs)

Pop-Tart Substitute

Nature's Warehouse "Pastry Poppers" (no refined sugar, good fats, no food dyes or preservatives; some are wheat-free for wheat-sensitive individuals)

Dairy Products (Protein)

Milk: AVOID THE BOVINE GROWTH HORMONE!!

Organic Valley (skim, 1%, 2%)

Horizon Organic Milk and Yogurt

Cascadian Farms (organic milk and yogurt)

Buttermilk (any brand, lowfat)

Oberweis (all dairy products; hormone-free)

Yogurt and Kefir

**The only safe dairy products are those that are certified organic or those that are imported from Europe (France, England, Italy, etc.) because hormone use for cattle has been banned in Europe

Stonyfield Farms nonfat yogurt (no refined sugars, many flavors, active acidophilus culture, delicious!)

Stoneyfield Farms "You Baby" full fat yogurt (in child size containers)

Cascadian Farms Organic Yogurt

Alta Dena Yogurt

Amish Yogurt (naturally free-range, hormone free)

Horizon Organic Yogurt (totally organic and fat free)

Lifeway Kefir (tastes like liquid yogurt; many flavors)

Brown Cow Yogurt

Milk and Yogurt Substitutes

West Soy Plus (fortified to duplicate the nutrients in milk)

West Soy Lite (lower in fat and calories)

Pacific Foods of Oregon Almond non-dairy beverage (fortified with A, D, Calcium, B vitamins, and Zinc; contains no barley malt)

Pro Soya So Nice Soy beverage

Rice Dream (plain, almond, vanilla, carob, and chocolate flavors; one variety is calcium-fortified)

Soya Latte (delicious yogurt substitute made from organic soy beans; contains an active yogurt culture)

Soy Dream (least allergenic)

Edensoy

White Wave Dairyless Yogurt/Silk Soy Beverage

Amazake Rice Nog (made from organic brown rice and almond sweetener) great for kids with food allergies who need fat, extra protein (11% per serving), extra iron (8% per serving), and B-vitamins . . . 272 calories per serving; (tastes good by itself or over cereal)

Cheese (Dairy) SEE "ANIMAL PROTEIN FOODS"

Animal Protein Foods
Red Meat

Kohler Pure Lean Beef (25-35% leaner)

Limousine Supreme Beef (no antibiotics, additives, or preservatives; less calories and cholesterol than chicken)

Laura's Lean Beef

Oberweis or Tamaso Beef (antibiotic and hormone-free)

Ostrich; very lowfat (3 gm. per serving); high iron; tastes like beef

Coleman Beef (antibiotic and hormone-free; tasted delicious)

Poultry

Harrison's Free-Range Poultry (chicken, turkey, turkey burgers, etc.; tastes delicious; sell to stores or their own store located on Waukegan Road in Glenview)

Phil's Range-Fed Poultry

Case Farms Poultry (from Amish Farms; antibiotic and hormone-free, no harmful chemicals used in cleaning)

Empire Kosher Poultry (no harmful residues)

Cornish Hen (most brands contain no harmful residues)

Duck (most brands contain no harmful residues; fatty - prick skin repeatedly while baking to remove excess fat and make duck crispier)

Eggs
Phil's Range Fed
Nest Eggs (antibiotic and hormone-free)

any brand that is free range and antibiotic/hormone free

Egg Substitutes
Jolly Joan Egg Replacer
Energ-G egg substitute

Make your own: 1 tsp. baking powder or 1 T. gelatin dissolved in hot liquid for each egg called for in recipes

Cheese (Dairy):
The only safe cheeses are those that are organic or imported (antibiotic/ hormone free)

Part-skim Mozzarella Cheese (low-in-fat)
Lifeway Farmer's Cheese
Farmer's Cheese (low-in-fat)
Pot Cheese (low-in-fat)
Low Fat Ricotta Cheese (dry curd cottage cheese can be used as a substitute)
Breakstone's cottage cheese (now comes in snack size packs)

Amish Yogurt Cheese (many flavors)
higher in fat varieties:
  Edam/Gouda/Havarti/Alpine
  Lace/Lorraine Swiss
Bravissimo All Natural Rising Pizza (finally a totally organic pizza without whole wheat flour!)
Alta Dena

Cheese Substitutes
Vermon Impastata creamy goat's milk cheese
Soyco Soy Cheese (these do have casein, dairy protein, so AVOID
Soya Cass Cheese if allergic to dairy products)
Tofu (can substitute for ricotta or cottage cheese in recipes)
VeganRella (finely a 100% non-dairy, no casein, no soy, cheese subsitute made from brown rice milk; available in mozzarella and cheddar flavors)

Non-Animal Protein Foods
Planters unsalted roasted peanuts
Real Brand Peanut Butter (found in the dairy case)
Smucker's all natural Peanut Butter
Tahini (sesame butter)
Pecan, almond, or cashew butter

David's Sunflower Kernels
Evon's Nuts/Seeds
Klein's Natural dried nuts and fruits
Nuts and Seeds (found in the bakery section, they most often contain no added fats or sodium)

Beans (Legumes)
Tofu (preferably organic, found in produce section; great in spaghetti, stir-fries, chili, or fruit shakes/sorbets) WHITE WAVE IS GREAT!
Reduced Fat Tofu from White Wave, Inc. of Boulder, Colorado (organic and lowfat)
Casbah Hummus and Bean Meals (easy-to-prepare)

Lundberg Pilafs
Soyco or Soya Cass soy cheese
Aunt Patsy's Pantry Lentil Chili
Jaclyn's Grilled Tofu and Bean Sauce (natural answer to a T.V. Dinner; with rice & veggie)
Boca Burgers (delicious; high soy, some with dairy protein; lowfat or no fat; no MSG derivatives)

High Protein Grains

Quinoa (plain for rice substitute or cooked cereal, pasta - avoid if corn sensitive)

Amaranth (cereal, plant or flour)

Mother's Quick Cooking Barley (use as a rice substitute or in soups)

Midland Harvest Burger 'n Loaf (no MSG)

Lundberg Pilafs (those containing beans)

Pure Protein Powders

GeniSoy Protein Shake (also offers Fat-Free Soy Protein Powder, not the bars)

Gam Octa Pro (soy) (Biotics Research Corp. Houston, TX - 25gm. protein per serving!!)

Nurtribiotic Rice Protein (great for allergic individuals) Fish (Animal Protein)

Fish

Chicken of the Sea Diet Tuna (no MSG derivatives)

Bumblebee Diet Low Salt Tuna (no MSG derivatives)

Sardines (any brand in tomato, mustard, or olive oil sauce)

canned salmon (any brand); rinse off excess sodium

Fresh fish (avoid most lake fish; farm-raised salmon, salmon-trout, and golden tilapia are usually chemical-free)

Star-Kist Naturally Low Salt, Low Fat Chunk Light Tuna (albacore in nothing except pure distilled water)

Homarus, Inc.Smoked Salmon (NO NITRATES)

Tel Aviv Kosher (Dempster,Skokie) has hand-cut Nova lox that are nitrate-free

Processed Meats (Animal Protein)

**Most processed meats are extremely high in fats and sodium. They also often contain MSG derivatives, sodium nitrites, added sweeteners, and food dyes. They should be avoided as much as possible.

Shelton's Turkey Sausage

Jones "Less Fat" Pure Pork Sausage (lower fat than most commercial brands, no harmful additives, tastes great especially if baked instead of fried)

Jones ham and Canadian Bacon (may contain a small amount of nitrates)

The Pork Schop of Vermont (uncured beef frankfurters or bratwurst)

imported baked or boiled ham (usually very low in fat, may contain nitrates, however)

lean turkey or chicken breast (avoid brands containing dextrose or nitrites) (See Deli Section)

Boar's Head Deli Meats

Pure Farms (all natural) Chicken Weiners

Soups

Walnut Acres (includes a wide variety of soups and broth; avoid the Chicken Broth, however; it contains MSG derivatives)

Perfect Addition Rich Stocks (chicken, beef, fish,and vegetable varieties); delicious frozen concentrates to make your own soups or enhance flavors of any recipes that call for broth or stock

Health Valley Fat Free Soups (all vegetarian and Chili appear to be free of MSG derivatives); they don't all taste great but can certainly enhance the flavor of your homemade soup and make it go farther.

Tabatchnick Frozen Bean Soups (Split Pea, GREAT! Northern bean, Minestrone, etc.; Contain no MSG)

Chef Earl's Soups/Sauces (vegetarian; no dairy)

Taste Adventure "instant meals" (many bean soup varieties; avoid the Red Bean Chili because it contains textured soy protein, a derivative of MSG)

Aunt Patsy's Bean Soups (they take a long time to prepare, but are delicious)

Fats/Oils
A good rule-of-thumb to keep fat content low is no more than 2 T. added fat daily (other than what is found naturally in breads/grains, meats/beans and vegetables)

rice bran oil,
small amounts of:
   Dynasty Sesame Oil
   Avocado Oil (tastes like butter)
   expeller pressed soybean oil
   expeller pressed peanut oil
   expeller pressed safflower oil

any brand of extra virgin olive oil
any brand of canola oil
Flaxsed oil (great source of Omega 3 fatty acids, great for digestion)
Flora cold pressed oils

Cooking Sprays
Weight Watcher's Cooking Spray (made with canola oil; doesn't contain flurocarbons)

Bertoli Olive Oil Spray (safe for environment)

Butter/margarine:
Hain Safflower Oil Margarine
Natural by Nature organic whipped butter (delicious!)
Promise Ultra or Smart Beat (canola oil)
any brand organic butter (Organic Valley)

better butter: use 8 oz. whipped butter with ¼ c. canola oil; whip together with a fork when the butter softens, can store in the refrigerator for 1 month
Spectrum Naturals (non-hydrogenated) margarine

Mayonnaise
Hellmann's Cholesterol Free Mayonnaise (does not contain egg yolk, does contain sugar)
for less fat and calories, mix mayo with nonfat plain yogurt

Soy Mayonnaise (with no added artificial ingredients)
good mayonnaise substitute: AVOCADO

Sour cream/cream cheese (not for dairy sensitive)
Breakstone's Light Choice (33% less fat)
light cream cheese - Neufchatel cheese - no fat (Philadelphia)

nonfat yogurt (organic) - sour cream substitute

Condiments
Vinegar
balsamic
rice wine
apple cider

gourmet-most types (especially brands imported from Italy)
vinegar substitute: lemon juice (fresh)

Spices/Salt
Sea Salt (salt with added minerals)
Vegit
Parsley Patch (no salt) seasonings (many varieties taste delicious)

Select Origins salt-free spices
fresh lemon juice or balsmic vinegar gives foods a salty taste naturally

Seasonings and Sauces
Lawry's Chili Seasoning Mix
San-J Tamari Lite (low sodium, no wheat)
most brands of mustard are O.K.
San-J Teriyaki Sauce (great marinade,
    no wheat)
Farmer's & Sittler's Horseradish164
Garlic Plus Chunky Garlic Onion Sauce
    (great for pasta, fish, chicken, steak)

Lea & Perrin Worcestershire (does con-
    tain a small amount of corn sugar)
Muir Glen catsup
Season's catsup (corn-free)
Westbrae unsweetened catsup
Grey Poupon Dijon Mustard (or any
    high quality mustard)

Salsa
Hot Cha Cha
Pace
Enrico's

Desert Rose
Ultima

Pasta Sauces
Classico Tomato and Basil Sauce
Classico spicy red Pepper Sauce
Enrico's
Silver Palate Sauce
Bertagni Basil Sauce
Ferrara Sauce
Romance Napole Sauce (refrigerator
    section, some have saturated fats)
Bartone Red and White Clam Sauce

Contadina Plum Tomato & Marinara
    Sauces (refrigerator section, some
    have saturated fats)
Progresso Red Clam Sauce
Pomi Marinara Sauce
Muir Glen (organic sauce)
Gianotti's sauce - delicious!
Tree of Life (organic)

Oriental Sauces
Hot Pepper Sauce (most brands are O.K.)
black strap molasses (high in minerals)

pickled ginger
miso paste

Salad Dressing
Higher-in-fat varieties
♦Higher-in-sodium varieties*

Brianna's homemade Dressings
*Lisa Jardine's Hill Country French
*Paul Newman's Olive Oil & Vinegar
*Bernstein's (many varieties)
*Cardini's Pesto Pasta (no vinegar) and
    Zesty Garlic (great for marinades);
    Lemon Herb (no vinegar)
Cook's Classic Oil-Free Marinades and
    Dressings
*Fast and Fabulous Dressing and
    Marinade
♦Select Seasonings dressings (delicious
    and nutritious answer to Good
    Season's - NO MSG)
Pritikin No Oil Dressings
♦Walden Farms Reduced Calorie Italian

Walden Farms No Fat dressings (many
    varieties);Ranch with sun-dried
    tomato is delicious
*Silver Palate dressings (delicious-taste
    like homemade); Lemon Splash and
    Caesar varieties are fabulous
Annie's Naturals

Tip: You'll use less of any dressing if you
pour it into a spray bottle and spray a
small amount onto your salad.

Great Homemade Dressing: Use a dash
of olive oil and a dash of your favorite
vinegar or fresh lemon juice. Add a
sprinkle of dried garlic, dried Italian
Herbs, or parmesan or asiago cheese for
added flavor.

Non-Dairy Hot Drinks

De-caffeinated coffee (very acidic; use only water-processed verieties)

Kuhn's Deli carries a low-acid coffee

Starbuck's Caffe Verona (low-acid coffee)

organic coffee (California Sunrise)

Coffee substitutes

cereal grain coffees such as Postum, Pero, Roma, or Bambuu (may need to avoid if grain-allergic)

Teeccino herbal coffee (caffeine-free, many flavors)

Calli whole food beverage (tastes like tea; gives you the lift of coffee without the side effects)

barley tea (tastes like coffee if very strong; great for alleviating constipation and other digestive problems)

Tea

Kaffree Tea (no caffeine, tastes the most like regular tea)

Black or black and green tea blends (Lipton, Bigelow, Tetley, etc.)

Herbal teas such as Lipton, Celestial Seasonings, Bigelow, Good Earth and Now Foods (avoid herbal teas if pollen, grain, or yeast sensitive)

"Alvita" (individual choices) tea (great for allergenic people)

Chinese green tea (strengthens immune system)

Essiac tea (strengthens immune system)

Women's Liberty Tea (great for hormone balance) by Traditional Medicinals

Smooth Move Tea (herbal laxative) by Traditional Medicinals

Cocoa

Droste's or Hershey's unsweetened cocoa powder (stir into hot milk or Rice Dream and add 1 tsp. pure maple syrup - dry cocoa is a delicious, lowfat substiute for baker's chocolate in recipes)

Carob powder (chocolate substitute; use as above in cocoa recipe)

Non-Dairy Drinks - Cold

mineral waters- many are flavored; no calories Evian, Poland Spring, Thorspring (no carbonation), Perrier, la Croix, Crystal Geyser with Vitafort (carbonated); Glaceau Fruit Water soda pop substitutes: Everfresh, Sundance Sparklers, Crystal Geyser Juice Squeeze, Knudsen Non-Alchoholic Spritzers (all contain fruit juice and sparkling mineral water – buy in preferably in glass to avoid aluminum in cans).

homemade spritzers - use any 100% fruit juice and sparkling mineral water; mix together in a 4:1 ratio

natural soda pop - still high sugar, but no harmful food dyes or preservatives; avoid if corn sensitive

Corr's Natural Soda, Sprite, Seven Up, Gingerale "super juice," preferably in glass containers.

Speas Farms "Parent's Choice" drink boxes (100% RDA for Vitamin C, 20% calcium)

Dole Paradise Fruits (from concentrate); aids in digestion; less acidic than orange juice

calcium-fortified orange juice (each 8-oz. glass contains the equivalent of an 8-oz. glass of milk; easier to digest and absorb than most milk or orange juice)

Knudsen Papaya Nectar (contains enzymes for digestion; very high in beta carotene)

Ferraro's Carrot Juice (comes frozen; organic; loaded with beta carotene; delicious)

Non-Dairy Drinks - Cold

Santa Cruz organic fruit juices (convenient for kids in drink boxes; delicious; fabulous and healthy lemonade)

After-the-Fall juice (delicious)

Lorina's sparkling lemonade (all natural, no corn sweeteners); imported from France

sports drinks- a natural answer to Gatorade

Twin Lab Hydra Fuel

any fresh orange juice

Knudsen Recharge

Mountain Sun juice

Baby/Toddler Foods and Infant Formulas

Earth's Best Baby Foods (organic)

Growing Healthy Baby Food (frozen, tasty)

organic juice (many brands and varieties)

"My Own Meals" (O.K. if the other choice is fast food!)

Healthy Times Arrowroot Cookies

Gerber organic baby foods

Beechnut, Gerber, & Heinz (choose only those with no added sugar, preservatives, etc.)

Ross Carbohydrate Free Formula (carbo must be added); for highly allergic or "Failure to thrive infants" (use only under the direction of a licensed health professional)

Mead Johnson "Infalyte" oral electrolyte replacement (very low allergy and digestible; rice-based)

"Cookies for Toddlers" - Healthy Times (wheat-free) Arrowroot cookies and Teething biscuits

Many large grocery stores today carry organic and "health" foods. In addition, we are very excited about the opening of large natural foods markets that have opened nationwide. We also have names of several farms that deliver organic items or specialty foods directly to your home. They include:

CASCADIAN FARMS
Rockport, WA (206)855-0100
Many delicious frozen organic products (vegetables, fries, frozen yogurt, sorbet, etc.)

DOUBLE "Y" CATTLE COMPANY
Libertyville, Illinois
(847) 362-8847
They deliver antibiotic-hormone free beef directly to your home. Their beef is lowfat and delicious!

ENER-G-FOODS
Seattle, WA
(1-800-331-5222)
Mail Order Breads; Grains that are allergy & gluten-free; great for celiacs and those allergic to wheat.

TIMBER CREEK FARMS
P.O. Box 606
Yorkville, IL 60560-0606
(630) 553-2208
Fax # (630) 553-1557
Timber Creek's Motto is "We Bring Safe Food to Homes." They deliver all over the Chicago area. All of their foods are organic and include meats, poultry, soups, salads, vegetables, fruits, grains, yogurt, tofu, etc. If you want safe food and don't want to shop for it, this is the place for you!

WHOLE FOODS MARKET
For a list of locations nationwide, contact their corporate headquarters in Austin, Texas at (512) 477-4455.

WILD OATS MARKET
For a list of locations nationwide, contact their hotline at 1-800-494-WILD or their website at www.wildoats.com.

REFERENCES

Chapter 2
Food additive information

Blaylock, Russell, M.D. *Excitoxins: The Taste That Kills*. Santa Fe: Health Press, 1994.

Buist, Robert, PhD. *Food Chemical Sensitivity*. New York: Avery Publishing, 1988.

Center for Science in the Public Interest (1501 16th Street, N.W., Washington, D.C., 20036-1499); Posters, Books, *Nutrition Action Healthletter*, Tapes, etc.

Food Additive Toxicology. Ed: Maga and Tu. New York: Marcel, Dekler, Inc., 1995. between Center for Science references and Hunter, Beatrice Trum

Hunter, Beatrice Trum. *Consumer Beware!* and *The Great Nutrition Robbery*. New York: Charles Scribner's Sons, 1976 and 1978.

Mindell, Earl. *Unsafe at Any Meal*. New York: Warner Books, 1987.

McGee, Charles, M.D. *How to Survive Modern Technology*. New Cannan: Keats, 1979.

Neurotoxicity: Identifying and Controlling Poisons of the Nervous System. Washington, D.C.: U.S. Congress, Office of Technology Assessment, U.S. Government Printing Office, April 1990.

LeRiche, W. Harding. *A Chemical Feast*. New York: Facts on File Publications, 1982.

Winter, Ruth. *A Consumer's Dictionary of Food Additives*. New York: Crown, 1984.

Wolfe, Sydney M., M.D., Editor. *The Public Citizen Health Research Group Health Letter* (monthly newsletter on health and food-related issues); 2000 P Street, N.W., Washington, D.C., 20036-1499.

Chapter 4
Protein References

Abraham, Guy. "The Calcium Controversy." *J. of Applied Nutrition*. 34 (1982): 69.

Abrams, G. E., et al. "A Total Dietary Program Emphasizing Magnesium Instead of Calcium." *J. of Reproductive Medicine*. 35 (5) (1990): 503-07.

Balch. *Prescription for Nutritional Healing*. 2nd edition. New York: Avery Publishing Group, 1997.

Carper, Jean. *Total Nutrition Guide*. New York: Bantam Books, 1987.

Cohen, Mark Nathan. *Health and the Rise of Civilization*. New Haven and London: Yale University Press, 1989.

D'Adamo, P. J. *Eat Right for Your Type*. New York: P. C. Putnam & Sons, 1996.

Eades, Michael, M. D. and Eades, Mary, M. D. *Protein Power*. New York: Bantam Books, 1996.

Eaton, S. Boyd, M. D., et al. *The Paleolithic Prescription*. New York: Harper & Row, 1988.

Gittleman, A. L. *Beyond Pritikin*. New York: P. C. Putnam & Sons, 1985.

Gittleman, A. L. *Super Nutrition for Women*. New York: Pocket Books, 1991.

Gittleman, A. L. *Your Body Knows Best*. New York: Pocket Books, 1996.

Page, Melvin, E. and H. Leon Abrams, Jr. *Your Body Is Your Best Doctor.* New Canaan, Conn.: Keats, 1991.

Degeneration-Regeneration. Biochemical Research Foundation. 1949. (reprinted by Price-Pottenger Nutrition Foundation, La Mesa, Ca.)

"Position for the American Dietetic Association: Vegetarian Diets." *J. of the American Dietetic Association.* November 1993, pp. 1317–1318.

Saltzman. *Amercian Journal of Clinical Nutrition.* 69:140, 1999

Schmid, Ronald F., N. D. *Native Nutrition: Eating According to Ancestral Wisdom.* Rochester, Vt.: Healing Arts Press, 1987, revised 1994.

Sears, B., Ph. D. *The Zone.* New York: Regan Books, 1995.

Werbach, Melvyn R. M. D. *Nutritional Influences on Illness.* 2nd edition, California: Third Line Press, 1993.

CHAPTER 7
References for Magnesium

Abraham G.E., G.E. "Premenstrual Tension." In: Leventhal M, ed. *Current problems in Ob Gyne.* Chicago: Year Book Medical Publishers, Inc. 1980: 1–48.

Abraham, G.E., Lubran M.M. "Serum and Red Cell Magnesium Levels in Patients with Premenstrual Tension." *Amer. J. of Clin. Nutr.* 34; Nov. 1981 pp. 2364–2366.

Abraham, G.E., et al. "Effect of Vitamin B6 plasma red cell magnesium levels in premenopausal women." *Ann. Clin. Lab Sci.* 11(4): 333–36, 1981.

Anast, C.S., et al. "Impaired Release of PTH in Magnesium Deficiency." *J. Chin. Endocrinol. Metabol.* 42:707, 1976.

Ashmead, H.D., et al. *Intestinal Absorption of Metal Ions and Chelate.* Springfield: Charles C. Thomas, 1985.

Ba, R.S., et al. "Hypomagnesemic hypocalcemia secondary to renal magnesium wasting." *Ann Int. Med.* 82: 646.

Barbeau, A., Rojo-Ortega, J.M., Brecht, H.M., et al. "Deficience en Magnesium et dopamine cerebral." In: Durlach J. First International Symposium on Magnesium Deficiency in Human Pathology. Paris: Vittell, 1973: 149–56.

Booth, C.C., et al. "Incidence of hypomagnesaemia in intestinal malabsorption." *BR. Med J.* 2: 141, 1963.

Caddell, J.L. "Magnesium in the therapy of protein-calorie malnutrition of childhood." *J. Pediatr.* 66: 392, 1965.

Ceriello, A., et al. "Hypomagnesemia in Relation to diabetic Retinopathy." *Diabetic Care.* 5; 558–9, 1982.

Cohen, L., Kitzes, R. "Infrared Spectroscopy and Mg Content of Bone Mineral in Osteoporotic Women." *Israel J. Med. Sci.* 17: 1123–5, 1981.

E. Whang, R., et al. "The influence of sustained magnesium deficiency on muscle potassium repletion." *J. of Lab. and Clin. Med.* 70:8950902 (1967).

Eliel, L.P., et al. "Magnesium metabolism in hyperparathyroidism and ostrolytic disease." *Ann. N.Y. Acid. Sci.* 162: 810, 1969.

Flink, E.B., et al. "Relationship of free fatty acids and magnesium in ethanol withdrawal in dogs." *Metabolism.* 28: 858, 1979.

Flink, E.B., et al. "Alterations of long-chain fatty acids and magnesium concentration in acute myocardial infraction." *Arch. Int. Med.* (In Press).

G. Shils, M.E. "Experimental human and magnesium depletion." *Medicin.* 43: 61–85 (1969).

Gersh, P.H., et al. "Symptomatic magnesium deficiency in surgical patients." *Ann. Surg.* 159: 402, 1964.

Goldman, R.H., et al. "The effect on myocardial 3H-digoxin of magnesium deficiency." *Proc. Soc. Exp. Bio. Med.* 136, 1971.

Hammarsten, J.E., and Smith, W.O. "Symptomatic magnesium deifiency in man." *N.E.J.O.M.* 256: 897, 1957.

Hirschfelder, A.D. "Clinical manifestations of high and low plasma magnesium." *J.A.M.A.* 102: 1138, 1934.

Holden, M.P., et al. "Magensium in patients undergoing open-heart surgery." *Thorax.* 27: 212, 1972.

Lindeman, R.D., et al. "Magnesium in Health and Disease." Jamacia, NY., *SP Medical and Scient. Books.* 1980, p.236–45.

"Magnesium Status by Acute Myocardial Infarction." *J. of the Amer. Coll. of Nutr.* Abstr#30, Vol.7, No.5, Oct. 1988.

"Magnesium Sulfate Reduces Mycocardial Infarct Size when Administered Before by not After Coronary Reperfusion in a Canine Model." Christensen, Carl, W., Ph.D., et al. *Circulation.* November 1, 1995; 92 (9): 2617–2621.

McCollister, R.J., et al. "Normal renal magnesium clearance and the effect of water loading, clorothiazide and ethanol on magnesium excretion." *J. Lab. Clin. Med.*, 52: 928, 1958.

Montgomery, R.D. "Magnesium deficiency and tetany in kwashiorkor." *Lancet.* 2: 264, 1960.

Nordin, B.E.C. "Plasma calcium and plasma magnesium homeostasis" In Nordin. BEC, ed Calcium Phosphorous and Magnesium *Metabolism.* NY: Churchill Livingstone, 1976.

O'Donnell, J.M., Smith, D.W. "Uptake of Calcium and Magnesium by Rat Duodenal Mucosa analyzed by Means of Competing Metals." *J. Physiol.* 229: 733, 1973.

Opie, L.H., et al. "Massive small bowel reaction with malabsorption and negative magnesium balance." *Gastroenterology.* 47: 415, 1964.

Paunier, L., et al. "Primary hypomagnesemia with secondary hypocalcemia." *J. Pediatr.* 67: 945, 1965.

"Prohylaxis of Migraine with Oral Magnesium: Results from a Prospective, Multi-Center, Placebo-Controlled and Double-Blind Randomized Study." Peikert, A. et al. *Cephalalgia.* 1996; 16: 257–63.

Rayssiquier, Y. "Hypomagnesemia resulting from adrenaline infusion in ewes: its relation to lipoysis." *Horm. Metabol. Res.* 9: 253, 1977.

Reinhart, R., et al. "Hypomagnesemia in patients entering the ICU." *Critical Care Med.* 13 (6): 506. 1985.

Rude, R.K., Bethune, J.E. "Renal tubular maximum for magnesium in normal, hyperparathyroid and hypoparathyroid Man." *J. Clin. Endocrinol. Metab.* 1080; 51: 1452–31.

Russell, R.I. "Magnesium requirements in patients with chronic inflammatory disease receiving intravenous nutrition." *J. Am. Coll. Nutr.* 4 (5) 553–58. 1985.

Scheinman, M.M., et al. "Magnesium metabolism in patients undergoing cardiopulmonary bypass." *Circulation.* 39: (Suppl) 235, 1969.

Schwartz, U.D., Abraham, G.E. "Corticosterone and Aldosterone Levels During the Menstrual Cycle." *Obstet Gynecol.* 45: 339–42, 1975.

Seelig, M. *Magnesium Deficiency in the Pathogenesis of Disease.* NY: Plenum Press, 1980

Thoren, L. "Magensium deficiency in gastrointestinal fluid loss." *Acta Chir. Scand.* (Suppl) 306: 1963.

Werbach, Melvyn R. M.D. *Nutritional Influence on Illness.* 2nd edition. California: Third Line Press, 1993.

Whang, R., Aikawa, J.K. "Routine serum magnesium determination—an unrecognized need." In Cantin and Seelig (eds) *Magnesium in Health and Disease.* pp. 1–5 (SP Medical and Scientific Books, NY, 1980).

Whang, R., et al. "Predictors of clinical hypomagnesaemia: hypokalemia, hypophosphatemia, hyponatremia, and hypocalcemia." *Archives of Internal Medicine.* 1984.

Whang, R., and Welt, L.G. "Observations in experimental magnesium depletion." *J. of Clinical Investigation.* 42: 305–313 (1963).

Wong,ET., et al. "A high prevalence of hypomagnesaemia and hypermagnesemia in hospitalized patients." *American J. of Clinical Pathologist.* 70: 348-352 (1983).

References for Calcium

Chan, G., et al. "The Effect of Dietary Calcium Supplementation on Pubertal Growth and Bone Mineral Status." *Clin Res.* 40: 60 A, 1992.

Chan, G., et al. "Bone Mineral Status in Childhood Accidental Fractures." *AJDC.* 138: 569–570, 1984.

Dixon, A. "Non-Hormonal Treatment of Osteoporosis." *Br Med J.* 286: 6370; 999–1000, 1983.

Durance, R.A., et al. "Treatment of Osteoporotic Patients, a Trial of Calcium Supplements and Ashed Bone." *Clin Trials.* 3: 67–73, 1973.

Epstein, O., et al. "Vitamin D, Hydroxapatite, and Calcium Gluconate in Treatment of Cortical Bone Thinning in Postmenopausal Women with Primary Biliary Cirrhosis." *Am J. Clin Nutr.* 36: 426–430, 1982.

Food Labeling: Health Claims; Calcium and Osteoporosis, Guide to U.S. Food and Labeling Law. Appendix III, 789–820, December 1991.

Heany, R.P. "Thinking Straight About Calcium." *N.E.J.O.M.* 328: 7; 503–505, 1993.

Johnston, C., et al. "Calcium Supplementation and Increases in Bone Mineral Density in Children." *N.E.J.O.M.* 327: 8287, 1992.

Mills, T.J., et al. "The Use of Whole Bone Extract in the Treatment of Fractures." *Manitoba Medical Review.* 45: 92–96 1965.

Pines, A., et al. "Clinical Trial of MCHC in the Prevention of Osteoporosis Due to Corticosteroid Therap." *Curr PrescrMed Res Op.* 8: 10; 734–742, 1984.

Reid, I.R., et al. "Effect of Calcium Supplementation on Bone Loss in Post Menopausal Women." *N.E.J.O.M.* 328: 460–464, 1993.

Riggs, B.L., et al. "Rates of Bone Loss in the Appendicular and Axial Skeletons of Women." *J Clin Invest.* 77; 1487–1491, 1986.

Stepan, J.J., et al. "Prospective Trial of Ossein-Hydroxyapatite Compound in Surgically Induced Postmenopausal Women." *Bone.* 10: 179–185, 1989.

Windsor, A.C.M., et al. "The Effect of Whole Bone Extract on Ca47 Absorption in the Elderly." *Age & Aging.* 2, 2300–2340, 1973.

References for Carnitine

Abdel-Aziz, M.T., et al. "Effect of carnitine on blood liquid pattern in diabetic patients." *Nutr Rep Int.* 29: 1071, 1984.

Bernsen, P., et al. "Successful treatment of myopathy, associated with complex I deficiency, with riboflavin and carnitine." *Arch Neurol.* 48: 334–8, 1991.

Canale, C., et al. "Bicycle ergometer and ethocardiographic study in healthy subjects and patient with angina pectoris after administration of L-carnitine: Semiautomatic computerized analysis of M-mode tracing." *Int J. Clin Pharmacol Ther Toxicol.* 26 (4): 221–24, 1998.

Cherchi, A., et al. "Effects of L-carnitine on exercise tolerance in chronic, stable angina: A multicenter, double-blind, randmized, placebo controlled crossover study." *Int J. Clin Pharmacol Ther Toxicol.* 23 (10): 569–72, 1985.

Carroll, J.E., et al. "Carnitine intake and excretion in neuromuscular disease." *Am J. Clin Nutr.* 34: 2693–9, 1981.

DiPalma, J.R., et al. "Cardiovascular and antiarrhythmic effects of carnitine." *Arch Int Pharmacdyn Ther.* 217 (2): 246–50, 1975.

Rossi, C.S., et al. "Effect of carnitine on serum HDL cholesterol: Report of 2 cases." *John Hopkins Med J.* 150:51–4, 1982.

Tripp, M.E., et al. "Systematic carnitine deficiency presenting as familial endocardial fibroelastosis: A treatable cardiomyopathy." *N.E.J.O.M.* 305: 285, 1982.

Trivellato, M., et al. "Carnitine deficiency as the possible etiology of idiopathic mitral valve prolapse: Case study with speculative annotation." *Texas Heart Inst J.* 11 (4): 370, 1984.

References for CoQ10

Baggio, E., et al. "Italian multicenter study on the safety and efficacy of coenzyme Q10 as adjunctive therapy in heart failure. CoQ10 Drug Surveillance Investigators." *Mol Aspects Med.* 1994; 15 suppl: s 287–294.

Bower, B.D., et al. "Treatment of idiopathic polyneuritis by polyunsaturated fatty acid diet." *Lancet.* 1: 583–5, 1978.

Folkers, K., et al. "New progress on the biochemical and clinical research on Coenzyme Q." In K. Folkers, et al., Biochemical and Clinical Aspects of Coenzyme Q, Volume 3. Amsterdam, Elsevier/N. *Holland Biomedical Press.* 1981.

Goldberg, A. *CFDIS Chronicle.* Summer/Fall 1989.

Judy, W.V., et al. "Coenzyme Q-10 reduction of adriamycin cardiotoxicity." In: *Folkers and Yamura.* Vol. 4, 1984.

Kamikawa, T et al. "Effects of Coenzyme Q-10 on exercise tolerance in chronic stable angina pectoris." *Am J. Cardiol.* 56: 247, 1985.

Kishi, T., et al. "Bioenergetics in clinical medicine. XI. Studies on coenzyme Q-10 and diabetic mellitus." *J. Med.* 7:307.

Kuklinski, et al. "Coenzyme Q10 and antioxidants in acute myocardial infarction." *Mol Aspects Med.* 15: s143–7,1994.

Langsjoen, P., et al. "Long-term efficacy and safety of coenzyme Q10 therapy for idiopathic dilated cardiomyopathy." *Am J. Card.* Feb. 15, 1990; 65: 521–23.

Langsjoen, H., et al. "Usefulness of coenzyme Q10 in clinical cardiology: A long term study." *Mol Aspects Med.* 15: s165–75, 1994.

Langjoen, P.H., et al. "Pronounced increase of survival of patients with cardiomyopathy when treated with Coenzyme Q10 and conventional therapy." *Int J. Tissue React.* 12 (3): 163–8, 1990.

Moricso, C., et al. "Effect of coenzyme Q10 therapy in patients with congestive heart failure: a long term muticenter randomized study." *Clin Investig.* 71 (Suppl 8): S 134–6, 1993.

Morisco, C., et al. "Noninvasive evaluation of cardiac hemodynamics during exercise in patients with chronic heart failure: effects of short-term coenzyme Q10 treatment." *Mol Aspects Med.* 15 (Suppl): s155–63, 1994.

Okuma,. K., et al. "Protective effect of coenzyme Q10 in cardiotoxicity induced by adriamycin." *Gan To Kagaku Ryoho.* 11 (3)L 502–08, 1984. (in Japanese)

Oda, T. "Recovery of load-induced left ventricular diastolic dysfunction by coenzyme Q10: echocardiographic study." *Mol Aspects Med.* 15 (Suppl): s149–54, 1994.

Saiki, I., et al. "Macrophage activiation with ubiquinones and their related compounds in mice." *Int J. Vitam Nutr Res.* 53: 312–20, 1983.

Shigeta, Y., et al. "Effect of coenzyme Q-10 in thyroid disorders." *Endocrinol.* Japan. 31: 755, 1984.

Shimomura, Y., et al. "Protective effect of Coenyme Q10 on exercise-induced muscular injury." *Biochem Biophys Res Commun.* 176: 349–55, 1991.

Van Gaal, L., et al. "Exploratory study of Coenzyme Q10 in obesity." In: *Folkers and Yamura.* Vol.4, 1984, pp369–373.

Wilkinson, E., et al. "Bioenergetics in clinical medicine. II. Adjunctive treatment with coenzyme Q in periodontal therapy." *Res. Commun Chem Pathol, Pharmacol.* 14: 715, 1976.

Yamagami, T., et al. "Bioenergetics in clinical medicine. VIII. Administration of coenzyme Q10 to patients with essential hypertension." *Res Commun Chem Pathol Pharmacol.* 14 (4): 721–7, 1976.

References for ACES

Burk, R.F. Letter. *J.A.M.A.* 262 (6): 775, 1989.

Burney, P.G.J., et al. "Serologic precursors of cancer: Serum micronutrients and the subsequent risk of pancreatic canc er." *Am J. Clin Nutr.* 49: 895–900, 1989.

Butturini, U. "Vitamins E and A in vascular diseases." *Acta Vitaminol Enzymol.* 4 (1-2): 15–9, 1982.

Combs, G.F., et al. "Can dietary selenium modify cancer risk?" *Nutr Rev.* 43: 325–31, 1985.

DeCosse, J.J., et al. "Effect of wheat fiber and vitamins C and E on rectal polyps in patients with familial adenomatous polyposis." *J. Natl Cancer Inst.* 81 (17): 1290–97, 1989.

Dieber-Rotheneder, M., et al. "Effect of oral supplantation with D-alpha-tocopherol on the vitamin E concent of human low density lipoproteins and resistance to oxidation." *J. Lipid Res.* 32: 1325–32, 1991.

Ferriera, R., et al. "Antixiodant action of Vitamins A and E in patients submitted to coronary bypass surgery." *Vasc Surgery.* 25: 191–5, 1991.

Fleet, J.C., Mayer, Jean, "Dietary Selenium Repletion may reduce Cancer Incidence in People at High Risk who Live in Areas with Low Soil Selenium." *Nutrition Reviews.* 55 (7) 277–9, 1997.

Freedman, A.M., et al. "Magnesium deficiency-induced cardiomyopathy: Protection by vitamin E." *Biochem Biophys Res Commun.* 170: 1102–6, 1990.

Frost, D.V., Lish, P.M. "Selenium in biology." *Ann Rev Pharm.* 18: 259, 1975.

Gey, K.F., et al. "Inverse correlation between plasma vitamin E and mortality from ischemic heart disease in cross-cultural epidemiology." *Am J Clin Nutr.* 53: 326S–34S, 1991.

Guo, W., et al. "Correlations of dietary intake and blood nutrient levels with oesphageal cancer mortality in China." *Nutr Cancer.* 13: 121–27, 1990.

Hong, W.K., et al. "Prevention of second primary tumors with iotretinoin in squamous-cell carcinoma of the head and neck." *N.E.J.O.M.* 323: 795–801, 1990.

Howe, G., et al. "Dietary factors and risk of breast cancer: Combined analysis of 12 case-control studies." *J. Natl Canc Inst.* 82: 561–9, 1990.

Knekt, P., et al. "Serum vitamin E, serum selenium, and the risk of gastrointestinal cancer." *Int J. Cancer.* 42:846–50, 1988.

Locktich, G., et al. "Cardiomyopathy associated with nonendemic selenium deficiency in a Caucasion adolescent." *Am J. Clin Nutr.* 52: 572–77, 1990.

McCarron, D.A., et al. "Blood pressure and nutrient intake in the U.S." *Science.* 224 (4656): 1392–98, 1984.

Moran, J., et al. "Dietary antioxidants and blood pressure-extended study." *Clin Res.* 39: A419, 1991.

Shklar, G., et al. "Prevention of experimental cancer and immunostimulation by vitamin E." *J. Oral Pathol Med.* 19: 60–64, 1990.

Singh, Vn., et al. "Premalignant lesion: role of antioxidant vitamins and beta-carotene in risk reduction and prevention of malignant transformation." *Am J. Clin Nutr.* 53: 386S–90S, 1991.

Stich, H.F., et al. "Remission of pre-cancerous lesions in the oral cavity of tobacco chewers and maintenance of the protective effect of b-carotene or vitamin A." *Am J. Clin Nutr.* 53: 298S–304S, 1991.

Werbach, Melvyn, M.D. *Nutritional Influence on Illlness.* 2nd edition. California: Third Line Press, 1993.

References for Lipoic Acid

Altenkirch, H., et al. "Effects of Lipoic Acid in hexacarbon-induced neuropathy." *Neurotoxicol Teratol.* 1990;12:19–20

Balch, James, et al. *Prescription for Nutritional Healing.* 2nd edition. NY: Avery Publishing Group, 1997.

Barzahi, N., et al. "Pharmacokinetic studies on IdB 1016, a silybin-phosphatidyl-choline complex, in healthy human subjects." *Eur J Drug Metab Pharmacokinet.* 15 (4): 333–8, 1990.

Constaninescu, A., et al. "Lipoic Acid protects against hemolysis of human erothrocytes induced by peroxyl radicals." *Biochem Mol Biol Int.* 1994; 33: 669–679.

Deak, G., et al. "Immunomodulator effect of silymarin therapy in chronic alcoholic liver diseases." *Ory Hetil.* 131 (24): 1291–2, 1295–6, 1990.

Greenamyre, J.T., et al. "The endogenous cofactors, thiotic and dihydrolipoic acid, are neuroprotective against NDMA and malonic acid lesions of striatum." *Neuroscience Letters.* 1994; 171: 17–20.

Guillausseau, P.J. "Pharmacological prevention of diabetic microangiopathy." *Diabete Metabol.* 1994; 20: 219–228.

Han, D., et al. "Alpha-lipoic acid increases intracellular glutathione in human T-lymphocyte Jurkat cell line." *Biochem Biophys Res Commun.* 1995; 207: 258–264.

Jacob S., et al. "Enhancement of glucose disposal in patients with type 2 diabetes by alpha-lipoic acid." *Arzneim Forsch.* 1995; 45: 872–874.

Jacob S. et al. "The antioxidant-lipoic acid enhances insulin-stimulated glucose metabolism in insulin-resistent rat skeletal muscle." *Diabetes.* 1996; 45: 1024–1029.

Kahler, W., et al. "Results of adjuvant antioxidant supplementation." *Z Gestamte Inn Med*. 1993; 48: 223–232.

Maitra, I., et al. "Lipoic acid prevents buthionine sulfoximine-induced cataract formation in newborn rats." *Free Radic Bio Med*. 1995; 18: 823–829.

Mascarella, S., et al. "Therapeutic and antilipoperoxidant effects of silybin-phosphatidylcholine complex in liver disease: Preliminary results." *Curr Ther Res*. 53 (1): 98–102, 1993.

Ou, P., et al. "Thiotic (lipoic) acid: a therapeutic metal-chelating antioxidant?" *Biochem Pharmacol*. 1995; 50: 123–126.

Packer, L., et al. "Alpha-lipoic acid as a biological antioxidant." *Free Radic Biol Med*. 1995; 19: 227–250.

Passwater, R. *Lipoic Acid: The Metabolic Antioxidant*. New Canaan, Ct: Keats Publishing, 1996.

Podda, M., et al. "Alpha-lipoic acid supplementation prevents symptoms of vitamin E deficiency." *Biochem Biophs Res Commun*. 1994; 204: 98–104.

Salmi, H.A., et al. "Effect of silymarin on chemical, functional, and morphological alterations of the liver. A double-blind controlled study." *Scand J Gastroenterol*. 17: 517–21, 1982.

Schandalik, R., et al. "Pharmacokinetics of silybin in bile following administration of silipide and silymarin in cholecystectomy patients." *Arzneim Forsch*. 42 (7): 964–8, 1992.

Schonheit, K., et al. "Effect of lipoic acid and dihydrolipoic acid on ischemia/reperfusion injury of the heart and heart mitochondria." *Biochim Biophys Acta*. 1995; 1271: 335–342.

Suzuki, Y.J., et al. "Lipoate prevents glucose-induced protein modifications." *Free Radic Res Commun*. 992;17:211–217.

Szilard, S., et al. "Protective effect of Legalon in workers exposed to organic solvents." *Acta Med Hung*. 45(2):249–56.

Thyagarajan, S.P., et al. "Effect of Phyllanthus amarus on chronic carriers of hepatitis B virus." *Lancet*. ii: 764–6, 1988.

Werbach, Melvin M.D., et al. *Botanical Influences on Illness*. California: Third Line Press, 1994.

References for B-Vitamins

Baker, AB. "Treatment of paralysis agitans with vitamin B6." *J.A.M.A.* 116: 2484, 1941.

Brattstrom, L., et al. "Impaired homocysteine metabolism in early-onset cerebral and peripheral occlusive arterial disease. Effects of pyridoxine and folic acid treatment." *Artherosclerosis*. 81 (1): 51–60, 1990.

Brattstrom, L.E., et al. "Higher total plasma homocysteine in vitamin B12 deficiency than in heterozygosity for homo- cystinuria due to cystathionine beta-synthase deficiency." *Metabolism*. 37 (2): 175–78, 1988.

Boers, G.H.J., et al. "Heterezygosity for homocystinuria in premature peripheral and cerebral occlusive arterial disease." *N.E.J.O.M.* 313: 709–15, 1985.

Clarke, R., et al. "Hyperhomocysteinemia: an independent rik factor for vascular disease." *N.E.J.O.M.* 324 (17): 1149–55, 1991.

Dalton, K., et al. "Characteristics of pyridoxine overdose neuropathy syndrome." *Acta Neurol Scand*. 76:8–11, 1987.

Ellis, F.R., et al. "A pilot study of vitamin B12 in the treatment of tiredness." *Br J. Nutr.* 30: 277–83, 1973.

Frank, O., et al. "Superiority of periodic intramuscular vitamins over daily oral vitamins in maintaing normal vitamin titers in a geriatric population." *Am J. Clin Nutr.* 30:630, 1977.

Kant, A.K., et al. "Dietary vitamin B6 intake and food sources in the US population: NHANES II, 1976-80." *Am J. Nutr.* 26 (12): 1339–48, 1973.

Kok, F.J., et al. "Low vitamin B6 status in patients with acute myocardial infarction." *Am J. Cardiol.* 63: 513–16, 1989.

Kopjas, T.L. "Effect of folic acid on collateral circulation in diffuse chronic arteriosclerosis." *J. Am Geriatr Soc.* 14 (11) 1187–92, 1966.

Keenan, J., et al. "Niacin revisted: A randomized, controlled trial of wax-matrix sustained-release niacin in hypercholesterolemia." *Arch Intern Med.* 151: 1424–32, 1991.

Lapp, C.W. "Chronic fatigue syndrome is a real disease." *North Carolina Fam Phys.* 43 (1): 6–11, 1992.

Manore, M.M., et al. "Plasma pyridoxal 5-phosphate concentration and dietary B-6 intake in free-living, low-income elderly people." *Am J. Clin Nutr.* 50: 339–45, 1989.

Parry, G.J. "Sensory neuropathy with low-dose pyridioxine." *Neurology.* 35: 1466–68, 1985.

Spies, T.D., et al. "Some recent advances in vitamin therapy." *J.A.M.A.* 115 (4): 292–97, 1940.

References for Saw Palmetto

Boccafoschi, S. "Annoscia S. Comparison of Serenoa repens extract with placebo by controlled clinical trial in patients with prostatic adenomatosis." *Urologia.* 50: 1257–68, 1983.

Carilla, E., et al. "Binding of Permixon, a new treatment for prostatic benign hyperplasia, to the cystolic androgen receptor in the rat prostate." *J. Steroid Biochem.* 20 (1): 521–23, 1984.

Champault, G., et al. "A double-blind trial of an extract of the plant Serenoa repens in benign prostatic hyperplasia." *Br J. Clin Pharmacol.* 18: 461–2, 1984.

Cukier, A., et al. "Permixon versus placebo." *C.R Ther Pharmacol Clin.* 4 (25): 15–21, 1985.

Duvia, R., et al. "Advances in the phytotherapy of prostatic hypertrophy." *Med Praxis.* 4: 143–8, 1983.

Emili, E., et al. "Clinical trial of a new drug for treating hypertrophy of the prostate (Permixon)." *Urologia.* 50: 1042–8, 1983.

Hanus, M., et al. "Alternative therapy of benign prostatic hypertrophy-Permixon." *Rozhl Chir.* 72: 75–9, 1993.

Mattei, F.M., et al. "Serenoa repens extract in the medical treatment of benign prostatic hypertrophy." *Urologia.* 55: 547–52, 1988.

Menendez, H., et al. "Use of amino acids as a combination in the treatment of prostatic hypertrophy." *Arch Esp Urol.* 41 (7): 495–9, 1988. (in Spanish)

Reece, Smith, et al. "The value of Permixon in benign prostatic hypertrophy." *Br J. Urol.* 58 (1): 36–40, 1986.

Tamca, A., et al. "Treatment of obstructive symptomatology caused by prostatic adenoma with an extract of Serenoa repens. Double-blind clinical study vs. placebo." *Minerva Urol Nefrol.* 37 (1): 87–91, 1985.

Vahlensieck, V.W., et al. "Benign prostatic hyperplasia–Treatment with an extract from the fruit of Sabal serrulata. A drug monitoring study involving 1, 334 patients." *Fortschr Med.* 18: 323–6, 1993.

References for The Algaes

Lee, William H., R.Ph, Ph.D. and Rosenbaum, Michael, M.D. *Chlorella.* New Canaan, Conn: Keats Publishing, Inc., 1987.

Rose, Jeanne. *Herbs & Change.* New York: Workman Publishing Co., 1972.

Woods, Rebecca. *The Whole Foods Encyclopedia.* New York: Prentice Hall Press, 1988.

References for B-12

Balch. *Prescription for Nutrition Healing.* 2nd edition. NY: Avery Publishing Group, 1997.

Berk, L., et al. "Effectiveness of vitamin B-12 in combined system disease." *N.E.J.O.M.* 239; 328, 1948.

Elsborg, L. "Vitamin B-12 and folic acid in Crohn's disease." *Dan Med. Bulletin.* 29 (7): 362–5, 1982.

Pagnelie, P.C., et al. "Vitamin B-12 from algae appears not to be bioavailable." *Amer. J. Clin. Nutr.* 53: 695–7, 1991.

Pennypacker, C., et al. "High prevalence of cobalamien (Vit. B-12) deficiency in elderly outpatients." *J. of Gerontology Society.* 8: A9, 1990.

Timiras, M. "Vitamin B-12 deficiency in geriatric clinic patients." *J. of Am. Gerontology Society.* 3898: A47, 1990.

References for Probiotics

Fernandes, Shahani, and Amer. "Control of Diarrhea by Lactobacilli." *J. of Applied Nutrition.* 40 (1), 1988

Fernandes and Shahani. "Lactose Intolerance and its Modulation with Lactobacilli and Other Microbial Supplements." *J. of Applied Nutrition.* 41(2), 1989.

Shahani, K., et al. "Immunological and Therapeutic Modulation of Gastro-intestinal Microecology by Lactobacilli." *Microecology and Therapy* 18:103–4, 1989.

References for Betaine HCL

Capper, W.M., et al. "Gallstones, gastric secretion, and flatulent dyspespia." *Lancet.* i; 4135, 1967.

(Abstract) "HCl deficiency amd chronic diarrhea." *J.A.M.A.* 39: 55, 1902.

Recker, R.R. "Calcium absorption and achlorhydria." *N.E.J.O.M.* 313 (2): 70–73, 1985.

References for Enzymes

Balch. *Prescription for Natural Healing.* 2nd edition. NY: Avery Publishing Group, 1997.

BioLinn, G., et al. "An evaluation of the importance of gastric acid secretion in the absorption of dietary calcium." *J. Clin Investigation.* 73: 640–7, 1983.

Lopez, D.A., M.D., Williams, R.M., M.D., Miehlkem. *Enzymes: The Foundation of Life.* Neville Press, 1994.

References for Ginkgo Biloba

Bauer, U. "Ginkgo Biloba extract in the treatment of arteriopathy of the lower limbs." *Pres. Medicale.* 15 (31): 1546–9, 1986.

Braguet, P., et al. "Ethnopharmacology and the development of natural PAF antagonists as the therapeutic agents." *J. of Ethnopharm.* 32: 135–9, 1991.

Chung, K.F., et al. "Effect of a ginkgolide mixture (BN 52063) in antagonizing skin and platelet responsed to platelet activating factor in men." *Lancet.* i: 48–51, 1987.

Kleijnen, J., Knipschildm, P. "Ginkgo biloba." *Lancet.* 340: 1136–9, 1992.

Kleijnen, J., Knipschild, P. "Ginkgo biloba for cerebral insufficiency." *British J. of Clinic. Pharmacology.* 34: 352–8, 1992.

Kunkel, H. "EEG profile of three different extractions of Ginkgo biloba." *NEUROPSYCHOBIOLOGY.* 27 (1): 40–5, 1993.

Markey, A.C., et al. "Platelet activating factor-induced clinical and histopathologic responses in atopic skin and their modification by the platelet activating factor antagonist BN52063." *J. of Amer Academy of Dermatology.* 23 (2): 2638, 1990.

Rai, G.S., et al. "A double-blind, placebo controlled study of Ginkgo biloba extract in elderly outpatients with mild to moderate memory impairment." *Curr Med Res Opinion.* 12 (6): 320–5, 1991.

Saudreau, F., et al. "Efficacy of Ginkgo Biloba extract in the treatment of lower limb obliterative artey disease of stage III of the Fontaine classification." *J. of Mal Vasc.* 14: 117–82, 1989 (in French).

Vorberg, G. "Ginkgo Biloba extract: a long-term study of chronic cerebral insufficiency in geriatric patients." *Clinical Trials Journal.* 22 (2): 149–57, 1985.

Wilkens, J.H., et al. "Effects of a PAF antagonist (BN52063) on bronchoconstriction and platelet activation during exercise induced asthma." *British J. of Clin Pharmacology.* 29 (1): 85–91, 1990.

References for Zinc

Bhattacharya, S.K., et al. "Significantly altered copper and zinc levels in serum, urine, liver, and skeletal muscle of morbidly obese patients." *J. Amer Coll Nutr.* 7 (5): 401, 1988.

Black, M.R., et al. "Zinc supplements and serum lipids in young adult white males." *Am J. of Clin Nutr.* 47: 970–75, 1988.

Bogden, J.D., et al. "Effects of one year of supplementation with zinc and other micronutrients on cellular immunity in the elderly." *J. Am Coll Nutr.* 9 (3): 214–25, 1990.

Fahim, M.S., et al. "Zinc treatment for the reduction of hyperplasia of the prostate." *FED PROC.* 35: 361, 1976.

Fell, G.S., et al. "Urinary zinc levels as an indication of muscle catabolism." *Lancet.* 1: 280–82, 1973.

Haley, J.V. "Zinc sulfate and wound healing." *J. of Surgical Residency.* 27 (3): 168–74, 1979.

Hallbook, T., Hedelin, H. "Zinc metabolism and surgical traumas." *British J. of Surgery.* 64: 271–73, 1977.

Hallbook, T., Lanner, E. "Serum zinc and healing of venous ulcers." *Lancet.* 2: 780–2, 1972.

Halsted, J.A., Smith, J.C., Jr. "Plasma zinc in health and disease." *Lancet.* 1: 322–24, 1970.

Henkin, R.I. "Zinc in wound healing." *N.E.J.O.M.* 29 (13): 675–76, 1974.

Mathe, G., et al. "A phase II trial of immunorestoration with zinc in immunodepressed cancer patients." *Biomedical Pharmacotherapy.* 40 (10): 383–85, 1986.

Newsome, D., et al. "The trace element and antioxidant economy of the human macula; can dietary zinc supplementation influence the course of macular degeneration?" *J. of the Am College of Nutrition.* 10 (5): 536, 1991.

Schrodt, G.R., et al. "The Concentration of zinc in diseased human prostate glands." *CANCER.* 17: 1555–66, 1964.

Silverstone, B.Z., et al. "Zinc and copper metabolism in patients with senile maculargeneration." *Ann. of Optham.* 17 (7): 419–22, 1985.

Umoren, J. "Serum total cholesterol and HDl cholesterol levels as associated with copper and zinc intake in physically active elderly men and women." *Advanced Experiments in Medical Biology.* 258: 171–81, 1989.

Underwood, E.J. *Trace Elements in Human and Animal Nutrition.* 4th ed. Landon: Academic Press, 1977: 198.

Wagner, P.A., et al. "Zinc nutriture and cell-mediated immunity in the aged." *International J. of Vitamin Nutrition Research.* 53 (1): 94–101, 1983.